BRAD GOUTHRO

THINK

and

LIVE

LEAN

**6 STEPS TO UNLOCK THE SECRET
MINDSET TO LIVE LEAN FOREVER**

www.LiveLeanTV.com

Gouthro, Brad
Think and Live Lean: 6 Steps To Unlock The Secret Mindset
To Live Lean Forever / by Brad Gouthro.
ISBN-13: 978-1519434418
ISBN-10: 1519434413

PRINTED IN THE UNITED STATES OF AMERICA

Book and cover design by Carolina Nava

Cover photo by Mai Tie Productions

First Edition

TABLE OF CONTENTS

ALSO BY BRAD GOUTHRO

AWAKEN THE ABS WITHIN
EAT CLEAN LIVE LEAN COOKBOOK
TEAM LIVE LEAN
LIVE LEAN AFTERBURN
LIVE LEAN 15
LIVE LEAN MELTDOWN
LIVE LEAN MASS
LIVE LEAN ABS
LIVE LEAN SPRINT

DEDICATION

I dedicate this book to each and every person who has inspired me to take risks, to live outside my comfort zone, and to realize that anything is possible. Jessica, my beautiful wife; you've changed my world and I'm so grateful to share the rest of my life with you! The late great, Napoleon Hill, thank you for enlightening me with your transformational words. My parents, Dale and Sheila; I couldn't have done it without your unconditional love and support. And last, but certainly not least, my brother Ian. The guy I idolized growing up. I'm so thankful to know you'll always have my back no matter what. Much love bro.

ACKNOWLEDGEMENTS

Most authors use this section to acknowledge their co-writers, business partners, editors, assistants, lawyers, agents, producers, and media team for creating the final product.

I would do the same thing, but my "entourage" is not quite as luxurious as that (yet). However, I do want to acknowledge my small, but hard working team that was directly involved with the creation of this book.

Jessica, my incredible business partner (and better half), thank you for always pushing me and making me feel like I can do anything.

Carolina Nava, my "I can help with that" book designer. I'm eternally grateful for your willingness to always offer help. You're a beauty.

I'd also like to acknowledge a few of the authors who have inspired me during my journey. Napoleon Hill, it's obvious your book, Think And Grow Rich, was one of my inspirations for writing this book. Also, Robin Sharma, Jack Canfield, Jim Rohn, and Anthony Robbins. Your philosophies have literally opened my eyes to what is possible and helped change my life. Thank you for your transformational words.

FORWARD

Change is absolutely inevitable! The one prediction we can make about you is that a year from now you will be different. You can decide where you want to go.
- JAMES W. NEWMAN

Brad and I first met about 2 and a half years ago. It was during a time in my life when I was "re-building" myself, my business, my body, and my love-life. I had been through a really rough decade, starting at the age of 18 when my brother and his girlfriend were suddenly killed by a stranger (we still don't know who), for no apparent reason. This tragedy devastated me emotionally, was the hardest time I've ever been through, and it certainly changed the course of my life. To keep a long story short, I struggled to find happiness, I lived for the moment not believing there would be a tomorrow, not understanding that I had anything to offer the world, and treating my life like a ticking clock. I stayed as busy as possible in New York City, with work, travel, friends and meaningless time-wasting activities.

Around age 28 I started to grow tired of this meaningless life. I wanted more. I wanted to help people and make a difference in the world. One thing I had been good at was getting in shape and helping others do the same. So I started seeking out people who were doing just that, but doing it on a larger scale than I was. To be completely honest, when I first found Brad it was by doing a simple Google search for "ebooks about Abs". His YouTube videos popped up and I was AMAZED. He had incredible camera personality, so genuine, so real, and so smart. He had a big following online and tons of testimonials from clients whose lives he helped change. I agreed with everything he said or showed about fitness and nutrition. He was also really hot. :)

Out of the blue one night, after obsessing over him online for a few weeks, I decided it wouldn't hurt to reach out and see if he would like to collaborate on a workout video with me. I saw that he had worked with another female co-host and thought it would be cool if we did a workout together. I honestly had no imagination of hanky-panky, honestly. What happened next was truly shocking: he wrote me back and said yes! This was the first time I had ever contacted anyone for a collaboration, and he had such a presence online I was sure he'd be too famous to even read my email. Anyway, the rest I guess is history, as we are now happily married and living our dreams together in Los Angeles.

What I want to say about this book is that it's about to change your life. It's not that it might, it's that it actually will. Whether you do the action steps or not, just the act of reading his words will affect you in a positive mood-lifting way. Brad is such an inspiration to be around. He has truly helped me change my life, find meaning, and help others, and I've been lucky enough to watch and support him as he changes the lives of hundreds of thousands across the globe. I'm telling you that I've been through hard times, I've felt what it's like to lose my "Why" and wander around this life without any purpose or drive. I whole heartedly believe every word that is written in these pages and I believe in your ability to take action on your own goals and start building the life of your own dreams one brick at a time.

Of course as you will learn later on in this book, showing up and taking personal responsibility for your own success is crucial, but it never hurts to give thanks and respect to those who have lighted your path along the way. Think of Brad as the guy with the flash-light in any of your life's dark storms that you go through. Stormy days are inevitable, but I hope you will come back to these words time and time again to help you find your way.

- Jessica Gouthro

INTRODUCTION

Whatever the mind can conceive and believe, it can achieve.
- NAPOLEON HILL

This was the quote that inspired my life transformation.

I've read hundreds of thousands of words from university text books, manuals, and self-help books, but nothing has stuck with me as much as those 10 simple words. In fact, I've learned more from those 10 words than 4 years of university study and thousands of dollars in tuition. This simple statement has literally helped me transform my life inside and outside of the gym.

With this book, it's my goal to teach you the steps I've used to change my life. You're going to learn how to take action on them and improve in all areas of your life. I call it the Live Lean Mindset.

But before moving on, I must clarify one thing. You may be asking yourself: *Does this mean all I have to do is sit on the couch visualizing and believing that I'm living lean?* Um, definitely **NOT**!

Although most people wish they could Live Lean, the question is, why do so few actually do it? I believe it all comes down to mindset. People fail to realize that Living Lean is not a race. It's not a temporary diet or 90 day workout program. Living Lean is a lifestyle comprised of habits that may be tough in the beginning, but eventually they become normal to you. This requires a serious mindset shift versus the, "get it fast, get it easy" instant gratification hype or the belief that people who are fit were just born with better genetics.

Trust me, this journey will take time. It will challenge you. It will require dedication. It will take willpower. You will have to sacrifice. You will need to push yourself outside of your comfort zone. But, I promise you, when you reach your goal, it's worth it. If you're reading this book, then it's likely there is a missing link keeping you from reaching your goals. That link is your mindset, and this book is about to change everything for you.

As you can probably tell, I am not one of those "new age" positive thinking people who believe all you need to do is just sit around wishing for things to come true. I consider myself a "positive realist". To add the Brad Gouthro "flavor" to Napoleon Hill's quote, I'd insert the following two words to the end, "… with action."

"Whatever the mind can conceive and believe, it can achieve…
with action."

As with anything in life, you must take massive action towards achieving your goals. I'm sorry to squash all the hype surrounding the mentality that all you need to do is visualize yourself losing weight. It just doesn't work. **To get anything worthwhile in life, whether it's to lose weight, build muscle, or find the love of your life, you must change the things you're currently doing, and work hard for it.** Since you already took action by reading this book, I'm confident you are ready to take responsibility for where you currently are in life, and are ready to take massive action towards changing it.

If that sounds scary, don't worry, I'm here to help. You are capable of extraordinary things in life, no matter what your current situation is. My job is to inspire you to take action on the steps in this book and create the extraordinary life you deserve.

And yes, when I say an extraordinary life, I'm not only referring to your health, I'm also referring to your personal relationships, your professional career, and your most important relationship, the relationship with yourself. I've become obsessed with trying to understand why some people can live a life of health and wellness, while others fail. I've learned it's much deeper than just exercising and working out. It's also about how you truly see yourself internally, your past experiences, your daily behaviors, and how you're letting them create your future.

Lets be real. It's not that difficult to Live Lean. The fundamentals are simple. Eat healthy foods and exercise your body. However, if it's so simple, why is 70% of the population out of shape, overweight, and obese? Well unfortunately the fundamentals are just a small piece of the overall puzzle. The real issue is the psychological limitations we place on ourselves. In order to permanently change and Live Lean, you must acquire the Live Lean Mindset. Every meaningful change comes from within. You must have the belief that it's possible to change. I used to say transforming your body was 80% diet and 20% working out. That may still be true for a "temporary" body. But to get the permanent body you've always wanted, I now believe Living Lean is 80% mindset and 20% fundamentals (i.e. eating healthy and exercising).

Once you make the required mindset changes discussed in this book, the fundamentals will become life long habits on auto-pilot. Living Lean starts with unlocking the mindset, followed by learning the fundamentals, then taking massive action. Without action, the knowledge of the fundamentals are pointless.

Now you may be thinking, *"But Brad, you're just a fitness, nutrition, and health coach. What is your background in psychology?"*

Let me say this. My background is from the School of Hard Knocks. I've been through things in my life that I never thought I'd ever experience. These experiences, which I'll share in this book, often cripple people mentally and leads them to live a life below their potential.

But I *chose* a different path. I share my personal experiences in hopes of making you realize that I am no different than you. I just made a series of *decisions* to make different choices based on the steps you will learn in this book. On the outside, my Live Lean Transformation Mission may seem like it's all about health. However I truly believe the same steps to master your health also apply to all areas of your life. Working out and eating healthy are the gateway to living your best life. The underlying message I teach on Live Lean TV, is about creating a better lifestyle through consistency, hard work, and action. It's about pursuing daily progress, not striving for perfection. The action-oriented steps found in this book transcend the walls of how to workout and eat healthy. We will touch on all aspects of how to create your best life, both physically and mentally.

So with that said, I hope you're ready to take this journey with me and get inspired to start taking action. I also hope you're open to the idea of potential failure. Yes, failure is bound to happen on this journey. Why? The reason is simple. Most people never take action on their goals because they fear failure. I know how that feels as I've often struggled with facing the big F. However, over the past few years, I'm learning the importance of embracing failure and seeing failure for what it really is. It's just an outcome. If it's not the outcome I was hoping for, I try to learn from it and move on. In 2012, I experienced a lot of outcomes that made it my most challenging year ever. Had I not "failed", I would have never learned from it, embraced it, and wouldn't be where I am today. I'm in a better place now because of those past failures. Had I not taken those risks, I would have definitely given up on my dreams of helping empower people to Live Lean. It's really scary to think of where I'd be in the world right now had I stayed in my comfort zone. Damn. Not a good visual.

If there's one thing I want you to take away from this book, it's this: ACTION. Knowledge alone does not make people successful. Successful results come from taking action on the knowledge. It doesn't matter how much knowledge you have if you never take action. Don't just read this book to gain the knowledge. Read this book and take action on the knowledge. Do something with it. The ability to take action in all areas of your life is what's going to get you results. Commit to whatever it takes to succeed. Living Lean is a lifestyle change, not a temporary diet. Having an "interest" in being healthy will only take you so far. Once you're truly ready and committed to making a lifestyle change, something just clicks, and success begins to happen.

Welcome to the beginning of your journey to Think and Live Lean. This journey is a simple one. However that does not mean it'll be easy. Simple and easy mean completely different things. Sometimes the simplest things in life are the most challenging. And that's what this journey will be. Always remember the wise words of Napoleon Hill, "there is no such thing as SOMETHING FOR NOTHING!". Whatever is of value in life cannot be obtained without a price. Now I'm not talking about a monetary price. I'm talking about the price of effort, commitment, and determination. But trust me, the price you pay in the form of sweat and discipline is far less than the value you'll get in your life from LIVING LEAN.

This journey will continuously challenge you to get out of your comfort zone and commit to taking *daily* action. It will be one of the most rewarding accomplishments in your life, and it all starts with that first step (and then the next step, etc). Every section of this book contains actionable steps to help you become the best version of you.

Also I want to point out that many statements and concepts will be repeated in this book. This was done on purpose for the benefit of your subconscious mind. Don't worry, it'll all be explained in simple, actionable, and fun ways in the upcoming chapters.

So I ask you now. Are you ready to create the Live Lean Mindset? Damn right you are. **Let's go.**

SECTION ONE
DESIGNING YOUR VISION

CHAPTER 1.1

FINDING YOUR WHY

He who has a why to live for can bear almost any how.
- *FRIEDRICH NIETZSCHE*

Imagine waking up every morning with a clear vision. An emotional purpose that inspires you to take action towards your goals every day. Not only do you wake up inspired to take action, but by the end of the day, you feel a sense of fulfillment as you move one day closer to Living Lean. That's my vision for you after applying the steps in this book.

It's incredibly important to first define your "Why" before beginning with the "What" and "How". When you are connected to your Why, you will be inspired everyday to take the necessary steps to create life-long healthy habits. That's the key to Living Lean. Creating daily habits that are set on auto-pilot. For example, when you brush your teeth at night, you don't think about it, you just do it. It's on auto-pilot. Trust me, once you find your Why, over time your daily healthy habits, such as working out and eating healthy, will become automatic. You will no longer have those internal debates whether to skip your workout and hit the drive-thru. Your Why will inspire and drive you to make the right choices that will bring you closer to your vision.

If you are working on something exciting that you really care about, you don't have to be pushed. The vision pulls you.
- STEVE JOBS

Here's an example of my life before finding my Why. After graduating with a business degree, I moved to Calgary, Alberta, Canada and felt like I was ready to take over the world of advertising. Unfortunately, reality smacked me in the face when I started applying for jobs with the best advertising agencies. I'd spend hours customizing my cover letter and resume to the specifics of the role. Then when I finally gained the courage to click that scary "Send" button, all I got was silence. Days, weeks, and eventually months went by without hearing anything. My journey to become the next Don Draper wasn't going to be as easy as I thought.

To pay the bills I was forced to take on various blue collar jobs. Now I have nothing but respect for blue collar workers, but this was not a life I thought I was destined to live. I worked in construction, I worked in landscaping, and I worked in a wood factory making Christmas reindeer. I was miserable. I eventually quit all these jobs and moved 2,400 miles all the way across the country to move back home with mom and dad and start over.

Even though I was crushed with a sense of failure, I kept hustling and eventually got hired as an Account Coordinator with an up and coming Advertising Agency in Halifax, Nova Scotia, Canada. It was actually great in the beginning. I remember receiving my first order of business cards with my name on them. Thanks to the "liquid courage", I felt pretty cool giving them out to girls at night clubs. Then that all came crashing down on me when I was talking to this particular cute girl at the bar. I told her I worked in advertising, may have overemphasized my role with the agency a little bit, and then proceeded to give her my card. Little did I know she ended up being my bosses sister. Huge fail.

As the months went on, I was beginning to realize working for someone else just wasn't for me. I would wake up in the morning unmotivated. I'd give myself just enough time to shower and shovel a bowl of cereal into my body. Then I'd sit in traffic waiting to go to a "job". It was also starting to bother me that I wasn't waking up feeling inspired nor was I going to bed feeling fulfilled. My two biggest accounts were a beer company and the lottery. Deep down I didn't feel good about enticing people to drink more alcohol or gamble their money away.

After two years I left the company to pursue another marketing job. Over the next 8 years I eventually worked with two other companies where I was faced with the same issues. I wasn't inspired, I had no purpose, and I didn't have any vision of what I wanted in life. I was missing my Why.

As I'll share in greater detail later in this book, I always struggled with self-confidence issues. A lot of this had to due with my insecurities with my body. Although I was an athlete growing up, I never took my training or nutrition seriously. I felt too uncomfortable going to the gym and pretty much ate nothing but bread. During the second half of this 8 year period of my life, I realized I needed to do something about it. I originally thought I'd build more confidence once I had more experience in the corporate world. Wrong. Being in a marketing role, I was responsible for a lot of presentations, client management, and other relationship building roles. Even though I was smart and had years of experience in the role, I still wasn't excelling. I remember the day when a co-worker with less experience was promoted over me. For a short period of time I was pissed off. Then I became enlightened. Eventually I figured it was time to start focusing more on building my self-confidence by working on my physical self. This change in mindset eventually led me down the path of finding my Why. Not only did I now have a vision for what I was looking to accomplish, I also had an emotional connection to why it was important to me.

I was now inspired to get up at 5am to hit the gym and was motivated to eat healthier. Not only was my body changing, but so was my confidence. So much so, all this new found confidence gave me the courage to eventually make one of the biggest and scariest decisions of my life. I decided to "fire my boss", become an entrepreneur, and teach the world how to Live Lean. I experienced how finding my Why changed my life and was now extremely motivated to help others find their Why through health and fitness. I truly feel once you overcome your inner battles and take action to transform your body, you gain the confidence that you can do anything in life.

I've now found the self-confidence that I was always looking for. I feel younger, healthier, and more energetic then ever. When I wake up every morning at 5am, I feel inspired. When I close my eyes at the end of the day, I now feel fulfilled. It's been an incredible ride and it all started with discovering my purpose.

Now that you've learned my story. It's your turn. I'm no different than you. I'm just doing different things. And those things are what this book is all about. So let me ask you a simple question. When it comes to your health and wellbeing:

Have you found your Why?

In other words, why do you want to Live Lean? Before reading any further, say your answer out loud right now.

I'm waiting.

Thank you for playing along.

Side note - *as you'll find out, this book is very interactive. It's not the type of book you just read. It's a work-along book where I'm expecting you to invest the time in answering the questions and completing the work* *as we go along.*

If you answered, "Because I want to be healthy" or "Because I want six-pack abs", you just gave me the same answer as 90% of the population. Unfortunately, that's not a good thing. Why? Because I'll be real with you, that's a weak ass answer that has no purpose or emotional connection to it.

Think about it. Is the answer, "I want to be healthy" going to get you off the couch to workout when you're feeling lazy? Is that answer going to motivate you to get out of bed in the morning to cook a healthy breakfast rather than hitting the snooze button and settling for a bowl of fattening cereal? Your Why and your purpose to Live Lean needs to have a deep emotional connection to it. It's needs to be powerful enough to motivate you to go to the gym at 4:30am and inspire you to cook that healthy meal after a long day of work.

> *When your why is big enough you will find your how.*
> *- UNKNOWN*

One of my mentors, Darren Hardy, made a really eye-opening analogy about the importance of creating a more powerful Why. His analogy went like this.

If I placed a 10-inch, 30 foot plank down on the ground and offered you $20 to walk across it, would you do it? Of course you would.

Now what if I placed that same plank across the top of two, 100 story buildings. Would you still walk across for that $20? Probably not. But what if I gave you a more emotional Why?

Here's an example of how I could do that. What if your kids were on the top of the other building and it was on fire. The only way to save them was to walk across the plank? Would you do it then? Of course you would.

So the question is, why would you not walk across the plank for $20, but you'd run across it immediately if your kids were in harm? The answer is this. Even though your risk of falling off hasn't changed, your Why has. In other words, your reason for wanting to do it has changed.

This is a classic example of when your Why is big enough, you will find your HOW. Are you starting to understand why it's critical to create a stronger, more emotional, and more powerful Why when it comes to your health?

One of the main reasons why most people don't get what they want is they haven't decided what they want.
JACK CANFIELD

Once you understand this and find your Why, it will get you through the tough times. And I'll be 100% real with you. There will be many of these tough times ahead. This includes finding ways to re-program your body and replace your poor lifestyle habits with new positive ones that will take you to where you need to be.

CHAPTER 1.2

CREATING YOUR GRAND LIVE LEAN VISION

Create the highest, grandest vision possible for your life,
because you become what you believe.
- OPRAH WINFREY

In the last chapter we worked on finding your Why. Now that you have created an emotional connection to why this Live Lean journey to is important to you, it's now time to get clear on your vision. Think about your vision as the destination to where you want to go with your health (and your life). Without this vision, every single decision you make and every single thing you do has no direction.

With a grand vision so much more can be accomplished since you have a GPS of where you want to go. You also become more resilient to short-term setbacks because lets face it, we all miss the occasional workout or eat the occasional bad meal. Without a vision you'd probably allow these temporary setbacks to stop all your progress. But with an emotional Why and a grand vision, you will always steer yourself back on path. Every setback doesn't have to mean failure. When you're determined to never give up, you will find success.

Getting specific with your grand Live Lean vision is a critical step to achieving the exact results you want in life. When you hold the vision, trust the process, and consistently put in the work, the results always happen faster.

If creating a Live Lean vision sounds overwhelming, don't worry. I'm going to share the exact vision that I created for my business back in 2012. Not only will I be sharing a lot of personal information about my Live Lean journey, but I'll also be sharing the journey I took with my entrepreneurial business. I'm doing this as it's my hope that my openness and transparency about my struggles will also help inspire you that anything is possible. As I mentioned earlier, 2012 was the most challenging year of my life from both a personal and professional point of view. It was the first full year of my entrepreneurial career as well as the year that my ex-wife left me.

Creating this vision helped me get clear on what action steps I needed to take to correct my failing business and move on with my life. Before having a vision, I continuously felt sorry for myself and blamed my ex-wife for leaving me during my lowest of lows. With the divorce I had to sell my less than 2 year old custom built house. This not only meant I didn't have anywhere to live, my personal training studio was also in the basement of my house. I had to sell all my brand new gym equipment, the dumbbells, the barbells, the squat rack, the rubber flooring, etc. Being a new entrepreneur, I was making less than $10,000 a year. This meant I didn't even think I had enough income to get approved to rent an apartment.

However as I see it now, my ex-wife did me the best of favors by leaving me. It helped spark my never give up persistence as I had no other option but to make my business a success. It also opened up the opportunity to meet my future wife (and business partner) Jessica. So it's my hope that sharing this personal vision with you will inspire you to do the same, no matter how helpless you feel right now. Having a clear vision can be the guiding light that answers all your questions on what to do next. After I share my vision, I'll take you through a set of specific questions to help you create your very own grand Live Lean vision.

My Business Vision (written in 2012)

It's 2017, Brad Gouthro Fitness, now known as Brad Gouthro Media Inc., is a highly sought after brand in the online and offline health, fitness, and nutrition industry. My passion and energy levels are the highest they've ever been, and I still have more to give. My 7 Secrets To Living The Lean Lifestyle message continues to spread internationally. Satisfied customers are proving that anyone can live the lean lifestyle as long as you consistently take action on my 7 secrets. The gym doesn't take over my customer's lives. In fact, they're losing fat and building muscle in less time since they follow the simple and efficient workout principles from my Awaken The Abs Within book. My customers also don't starve themselves. They actually eat more food and are losing more fat by following my TQT nutrition principles also found in Awaken The Abs Within.

This is what makes me, my product, and my message different. I take complex and often confusing topics, and make it simple, implementable, and sustainable for anyone. People are connected and drawn to me based on my simple message and because I'm also living the healthy lifestyle that I promote. I relate, connect, and inspire people, not just create and sell them. I outsource any tasks that I don't add value to. My employees love working on the business, believe in the message, and are also living the lifestyle. This includes a team of 3 passionate writers, an advertising agency, 2 customer service reps/assistants, and a team of professional consultants including a publicist, TV agent, and literary agent.

Awaken The Abs Within just sold its 100,016 copy online. It also was just re-published as a paperback by selling over 20,000 copies and growing every day. My products also provide over 20 affiliates with enough sales to have financial freedom. These affiliates are a part of a mastermind group that meets in a fun location at least once per year. My affiliates and employees are not just sales people, they are my partners and friends. We've just accomplished our first mission of transforming the lives of 10,000 men, women and families via our Team Live Lean membership community. The community and its content continuously grows everyday. Next mission? 100,000 members by 2020. But I don't look at Team Live Lean members as just subscribers. Each member is a part of a movement to a healthier society. Not only are my members getting incredible results, they're also sharing the message and helping others move their bodies more efficiently and eating higher quality food.

Our e-newsletter currently has 1,000,347 subscribers and is e-mailed out daily. I receive customer feedback everyday via blog comments, personal e-mails, tweets, facebook posts, etc., describing how my message and products has inspired them to live a healthier lifestyle.

Not only am I well known in the online publishing industry, thanks to various business partnerships, I also currently have six figure endorsement deals with a supplement company and an athletic apparel company. All brands that I respect and use myself.

I'm currently in talks with a major TV network to star in a healthy lifestyle show. Even with all this going on, I still speak at and attend health and fitness conferences to continuously spread my message and connect with other potential business partners.

Finally, here are the top 6 words most people use when talking about me:
"BRAD INSPIRED ME TO TAKE ACTION."…the rest is history.

There you have it. That's what I wrote in 2012. Since

then a few things have changed, but that's ok as your grand vision should be flexible. Overall the vision of inspiring people to Live Lean is still in tact, but my approach to getting there has slightly changed. Here are a few new additions based on the slight change in my vision from 2015.

My Updated Business Vision (from 2015)

The year is 2020. Our Live Lean TV media company is a thriving and trustworthy brand in the online and offline health and fitness industry. The growth of our brand has been rapid, yet we still have so much more to give. Not only has our reach grown substantially but we have also grown our internal team. Although we try to keep our business as lean as possible (no pun intended), we realize that in order to keep up with the growth, we need to invest more in the business by hiring talent to help us manage the growth. Here's an example of our success to date:

- With over 5 million unique visitors each month, LiveLeanTV.com is one of the top visited fitness and health websites on the internet. New articles are published to the site everyday. Our website staff includes an editor, 2 new writers, a web designer, an IT developer, and a product coordinator.
- With over 2,000,000 subscribers and 250 million views, Live Lean TV is one of the most subscribed and viewed fitness channels on YouTube. We upload new episodes 3 times a week. Our channel staff includes a videographer/editor, product manager, 1 new host, and product coordinator. We also own a 10,000 square foot production studio that includes a fitness set, a kitchen set, and an office for our staff.
- With over 10,000 members on our TeamLiveLean.com inner circle members site, we continually add new monthly workout programs and weekly cooking videos, meal plans, and grocery lists. Our staff includes a product manager,

product assistant, and customer support manager.

- We continually hang out with over 5,000,000 followers across all our social media channels. Our staff includes a social media coordinator.
- We also launch a new premium product to the marketplace every quarter.
- In addition to our staff, we also have a talent team including a manager/agent to bring in sponsorship/endorsement deals, a publicist to provide us with media attention, an attorney to structure our business deals, and an accountant to manage our finances.

These are the updates to my grand business vision. I share this with you because I look at you as being an ambassador and a shareholder in our success. When we win, you win.

My vision is not perfect, but it does guide my decision making. It gives me the framework to say yes to things that will take me closer to this vision, while saying no to things that don't. See how powerful creating your vision is?

CHAPTER 1.3

IGNITING YOUR BURNING DESIRE

The starting point of all achievement is desire.
- NAPOLEON HILL

Imagine what you could accomplish if you were committed to working towards your burning goal EVERYDAY. I use the word "burning" because your desire to obtain your goal needs to be so hot, no obstacles can put out that fire. I mean lets be real. Transforming your body and health can be a slow and discouraging process. This is why it's extremely important that deep down, you really want this. Your desire to transform needs to be so strong that you can overcome any discouragement and criticism from others. It'll push you past the disappointment of temporary defeat from "slow results". It will also give you an unfound sense of confidence when you're faced with consistent peer pressure from friends and family to just "be normal" and enjoy life.

Without a sense of urgency, desire loses its value.
- JIM ROHN

In essence, this burning desire must be so hot and urgent, that no matter what obstacles stand in your way, you'll overcome them. Here's an example from my life. Back in 2007, when I finally made the decision to transform my body, I thought I could do it alone. I remember thinking how hard could it really be. Lift a few weights, run on the treadmill, and eat low calorie foods. Simple right? Well, after many failed attempts, I realized I was in over my head and needed a coach. Big breakthrough. However the problem was I couldn't find any trainer at my gym that was getting the results that I wanted. I remember thinking, why would I invest my hard earned money with someone that wasn't living their message. I was extremely frustrated as my search hit a wall. Then one day when I was looking for some motivation, I sat down with my computer, opened Google, and typed in the search term "World's Best Body". The first image that appeared was the exact physique I wanted to accomplish.

This guy was lean, ripped, athletic looking, and was close to the same height as me. I then dug a little bit deeper to try to find out what his workouts looked like. With a little bit of searching, I came across his website and found out he offered coaching. As excited as I was, in the back of my head I knew there was a 0.03% chance this guy lived in my city. Then my instincts turned into reality when I found out he lived in Los Angeles. At the time I was living in Halifax, Nova Scotia which is on the east coast of Canada. So not only was I located on the other end of North America, but I was also on the other side of North America too. After digging a little bit deeper, I realized he offered something called "online coaching". Although online coaching is very common today, back in 2007 it was still in it's beginning stages. I remember wondering how could I be coached online on a topic that was so hands on like fitness? I was discouraged. Then when I saw the cost, my stomach sank. It was way outside my budget and comfort zone. I even had to pay the money up front which was especially scary since I was paying someone online that I never met before. This would have discouraged most people from pursuing this opportunity. But did I give up? Definitely not. I was determined to make it work. My burning desire to change my body and ultimately my self-confidence was so hot, I had no other choice but to overcome all of these obstacles. Long story short, I took a leap of faith, sent him the money, received the coaching, and worked my freaking butt off. The rest is history.

Same thing was true with my business. When I was starting my entrepreneurial career in fitness, I made less than $2.30 an hour. If that wasn't bad enough, I was also going through a divorce. Not only did I lose my best friend and biggest supporter, as I mentioned earlier, I also lost my brand new house and my personal training studio. I didn't have a pension anymore. I didn't have a steady stream of income coming in. And I wasn't even sure I could get approved to rent an apartment. Did I give up on my entrepreneurial dream and play it safe by going back to the corporate world. Hell no. By applying all the teachings that I'm sharing with you in this book, I was able to make it work and overcome all of these obstacles. When you desire something so deeply that you are willing to put your entire future on the line, you will surely win.

Now it's time to get into more detail about igniting your burning desire to Live Lean. In a previous chapter we talked about going deep to find your Why. If you haven't yet completed this exercise, stop reading and start doing. I'm serious. Write down your Why. This Why is what feeds your burning desire and makes it hot! Every successful person started off with a Why and a burning desire for achievement. If your goal is to Live Lean (or whatever your goal may be), it has to create such a burning emotional response inside of you, that you'll do anything to have it. This means it's not something you wish will happen. It's not something you hope will happen.

It's a goal that you are positively committed to making happen.

Miracles don't happen. Sweat happens. Effort Happens.
Thought Happens.
- UNKNOWN

Now don't get me wrong. My journey started as a wish and a hope. I wished I looked like that guy on the website. I hoped my online business would be successful enough that I wouldn't have to work a corporate job anymore. However, all the wishing and hoping never got me anywhere. One day I finally got serious and committed. I created a burning desire that sparked such an emotional reaction inside of me that I had no other choice but to take continuous daily action towards it. I fueled my mind with success conscious thoughts. I visualized what it would be like to work on projects that actually impacted people's lives in a positive way and worked my butt off. Failing was never an option. As the saying goes, I burned the ships once I arrived on land. I had no other option but to succeed. There was no going back. You must be willing to burn your Live Lean ship as well to ensure you don't have an escape plan. When you're challenged with tough times, it's human nature to follow the path of least resistance. But that path is not for achievers like you. What separates the winners from the losers is being able to overcome adversity and challenge.

Every time I wanted to give up on my entrepreneurial lifestyle, the thought of going back to a purposeless corporate job created so much pain inside of me that it made me sick. Now ask yourself, what's the pain you're going to experience if you don't accomplish your goal. Once you've figured that out, go back to that painful feeling every time you're about to give up. Because lets be real, thinking about giving up is inevitable in your journey to Live Lean. I know I did. They'll be times where you feel like your body isn't changing, you're stuck in a plateau, the people closest to you are encouraging you to go back to your old ways. But at the end of the day, you and your new Live Lean Mindset must overcome all these negative outside forces. You must continue to see in your mind the person you WILL become (not TRY to become). Keep taking action and commit to consistently working towards making exercise and eating healthy a lifestyle habit. Can you see how different this is than having a non-committed mindset of: "I'll give this workout program and/or diet a try for 4 weeks, and if it doesn't work, I'll just quit". No you won't quit. Burn the damn boat! There's no going back. That's the incredible power of having a burning desire. And that's the desire I used to transform my body and career.

Trust me. Once your goal becomes a reality, and it will, you'll feel a sense of accomplishment that you can do anything you put your mind to. But be prepared that once you do succeed, they'll be plenty of failure conscious people along the way that will say you were just lucky, or you were born with good genetics. I get this all the time. These are the people that aren't ready to change. They're not ready to commit to the challenge and step outside their comfort zone. If these thoughts of luck or "you were born with it" have crossed your mind, squash it at soon as possible. Celebrate others successes, think in abundance, and stay open to the real cause of their success: commitment, hard work, and persistent action towards achieving their goal.

I still have nights where I'm sitting on my balcony, looking out at the city skyline, and reflecting on how far I've come both physically, mentally, and professionally (it's actually nighttime as I write this on my balcony). Now I don't say this to brag. I say this because I'm proof, that everything I'm sharing with you in this book works, if you follow the teachings. I must add, I'm still on my journey. I still have many things in my life, professionally and emotionally, that I'm working on. But the major win of transforming my body physically was my green light. It's what gave me the confidence that I could transform any area of my life.

A question I'm always asked, and is often debated

amongst coaches, is should you share your goals with others? To be honest, I have mixed feelings. So much so, I just hosted a live Periscope to hear your feedback and experiences with it. If you remember being on that Periscope, high-five to you my friend. The feedback was mixed, but I would say the majority of you have chosen not to share your fitness goals with others. To be honest, I agree under most circumstances. As you begin your Live Lean journey, I caution you to be very careful when sharing your goals with certain people. Here's the reason. In the beginning you're very vulnerable and nothing will kill motivation faster than having someone close to you make fun or criticize your new lifestyle. When it comes to fitness, I see this all the time.

Here's an example. George is a 35-year-old account executive at an advertising agency. He notices his belly fat is bulging over his belt buckle more and more everyday, so he decides it's time to stop taking his health for granted. He tells his beer-drinking buddies (who are also experiencing the bulge) that he's going to invest in a workout and nutrition program to lose 20 pounds and keep it off forever.

What kind of reaction do you think George is going to receive from his beer-drinking buddies? More than likely, he's probably going to be ridiculed and poked fun of. I experienced this exact same feedback. Most of the time, these exact people who are dishing out the criticism are actually very self-conscious, unhappy, and lack the willpower to change themselves. This is often referred to as crabs in a bucket. It's a metaphor that describes when a bunch of crabs are placed in a bucket, if one tries to escape, all the others gang up on it and pull it back down rather then helping it succeed. Essentially it's the "if I can't have it, neither can you" mentality. Does this sound familiar amongst your friends and loved ones? If not, be grateful that you are surrounded with amazing people. Unfortunately most people that I've talked to are being pulled back into the bucket. Not only is it tough to share your goals and become vulnerable in front of your friends, it's even tougher when your vulnerability is faced with criticism and doubt from the people you're closest with. This typically leads to people like George to quit before he even starts working towards his goal.

Don't ever let somebody tell you that you can't do something.
- WILL SMITH (Pursuit of Happyness)

The quote above is one of my favorites. But I'm sure you'll agree with me that it's easier said then done. Unfortunately what others say can have a huge impact on your actions, especially at a time of vulnerability. Ultimately you have to make the decision of who you share your goals with. It's my hope that you have at least one supportive person in your life that will help push you to keep achieving. If not, you always have me. I don't say that to be cheesy. I mean it. I truly believe that every single one of you can adopt the Live Lean Mindset. Whether you have a solid support group or not, I challenge you to keeping believing and go after what you desire. Spend more time hanging out with like-minded people in person, or join inspirational online groups like our TeamLiveLean. com Inner Circle or my Facebook Page at Facebook.com/ BradGouthroFitness. There are supportive people out there. You just have to find them.

If you live long enough, you'll make mistakes.
But if you learn from them, you'll be a better person.
It's how you handle adversity, not how it affects you.
The main thing is never quit, never quit, never quit.
- BILL CLINTON

There are also an abundance of people that are going through the exact same experiences as you. I too have experienced, and still do to this day, temporary defeats in certain areas of my life. However, one of the big key learnings I've picked up along the way is this. I now view adversity and temporary defeats as the necessary seeds to success. I've read a lot of autobiographies of successful people and the one thing that is consistent throughout all of their stories is how they started slow. They faced many failures, they wanted to quit, and a lot of them hit rock bottom. But here's the difference. They had a burning desire inside of them that kept pushing them forward until finally reaching a turning point of success. Sometimes we're forced to hit rock bottom before discovering what we are really capable of. As a 32 year old man, not only was my heart crushed from losing my best friend and wife to a divorce, but my entrepreneurial business was a joke. I also lost all connection with my closest friends that I hung out with since I was 5 years old. I was completely lost both in my personal and business life. This downward spiral probably would have driven most people to alcohol or drugs. Fortunately for me, I've never used those things as crutches. My burning desire to succeed as an entrepreneur was so strong that I kept an open mind, stayed persistent, and used those setbacks as motivation to work harder. But don't get me wrong. There were plenty of times I almost gave up. That is when my persistence finally paid off. Just when I was about to give up, something just clicked. Out of the blue, I received a few lucrative business offers as well as a random e-mail from a female follower from California named Jessica. Yes, the same Jessica who is now my wife! Call it ironic, call it mysterious, it doesn't matter. What does matter is I remained persistent throughout it all, I didn't give up when times were terrible, and as hard as it was, I believed in my abilities even when the critics were telling me otherwise. Remember this. Your reactions to the challenges and obstacles you face are completely within in your control. You are never defeated until you accept defeat as reality. If I can do it so can you. If Thomas Edison can fail 10,000 times, I'm positive you can find the courage and guts to overcome a few defeats and continue pursuing your goals.

However, I don't want you to just set easy to obtain goals. Set higher goals and stretch yourself to reach them. Once again, the starting point to creating your Live Lean Mindset is to believe, not wish or hope. These are two completely different things. Wishing and hoping are close-minded and do not create action. Once you truly believe you will accomplish something, then and only then are you open and ready to receive it. In order to really believe you can accomplish something, you must first believe in yourself and your abilities. Secondly you must believe you truly deserve it. And third, you must have the courage to refuse to accept the possibility of failure. Top all of this off with persistent commitment to action, and you will turn your burning desire into reality. This has worked for so many "failure to success" stories. All success starts with an intense desire to achieve your goals. So I ask you, would you describe your desire to Live Lean as intense and on fire? If so, you're a success story in the making.

Our only limitations are those we set up in our own minds.
- NAPOLEON HILL

LIVE LEAN ACTION STEPS

It's time to take action and apply what you learned towards your own personal situation. If you're not committed, there's no point in reading any further. This is not a book where all you have to do is just sit back and read. Sorry. Being a passive reader will only get you so far. It should come as no surprise that I want you taking action on every principle in this book. That's why I wrote it. This book was the missing link in my portfolio of Live Lean programs. It's now ready for you to 100% act on. Do yourself a favor and complete the action steps at the end of every chapter before you continue reading any further. With that said, lets take action!

ACTION STEP #1: WRITE DOWN YOUR WHY

To help you get your emotional juices flowing, here are a few examples of a strong and emotional Why. But don't just pick one of these that you think may apply to you. Once again, your Why needs to be very personal, very emotional, and very customized to your desires. This is an extremely important step for the entire journey of this book. Spend some on this. Feel free to Tweet your Why to me @BradGouthro. I can't promise that I'll have the time to respond to them all, but if I do see it, I'll try to help you out. Deal? Ok, cool.

Questions To Help You Find Your Why:
1. How will Living Lean make you feel more alive? Become more passionate? Provide more value to others and the world? Become more influential? Become a better parent/lover/friend?
2. How will Living Lean help you pursue your passion with more energy and focus?
3. How will Living Lean help you leave a legacy after you're gone?

Find Your Why examples:
• You want to live with energy and strength so you can be

around to play with your grandkids.

- You want to re-ignite the physical passion you once had with your husband or wife.
- You want to transform your body to increase your self-confidence so you'd feel comfortable walking down the beach in a bathing suit any day of the year.

By now, I'm hoping I've sparked up some emotional feelings inside of you. If not, don't worry. It'll take some time and reflection to get deep and emotional. And that's where you need to be. That's where I went when I found my Why. I hit my breaking point and promised myself that I would not suffer anymore. I decided that I was no longer willing to accept living a life of low self-esteem and confidence. I was destined to be better than that.

Whatever your Why means to you, figure it out, write it down, and go back to it whenever you're feeling like giving up. Once you discover your emotional reason, then and only then will you do what is required to make it happen. There will be times when you skip a workout, when you eat a bad meal, when you feel like you failed and want to quit. But when you have your emotional Why, you'll force yourself to push harder because you'll always remember why you started in the first place.

ACTION STEP #2: WRITE DOWN YOUR LIVE LEAN VISION

It's now your turn to create your grand Live Lean vision. Here's what I want you to do. In your journal, on your computer, or where ever you write things, for the next 45 minutes get creative and write out your Live Lean Vision. I'm most creative with my writing when I find a quiet place that inspires me and where I won't be disturbed. Pour yourself a cup of coffee (the caffeine will help you focus), open up a window to hear nature, and play some inspiring music (Coldplay is my go-to writing music).

Here are a few guidelines to follow:

1. **Your vision should inspire and fire you up.** Write with passion.

2. **Write as if you've already accomplished it.** Envision what it will be like after you're on your way to Living Lean.

3. **Be very specific, clear, and concise.** If you close your eyes, you should be able to see it.

4. **It doesn't need to be perfect.** Review it occasionally and re-write any part that doesn't fit into your current vision.

Here are 6 steps to start writing your vision:

1. What body fat % will you have when you reach your goal? I prefer body fat % measurement (or waist size of pants) rather than a weight loss goal for numerous reasons. Your body composition is comprised of the amount of weight coming from lean muscle tissue and body fat. In other words, you'll see how much of your weight is made up of lean muscle mass vs. fat. It's a much better metric of success than just a weight scale. Therefore, for people who only need to lose a few pounds of fat, your weight may not fluctuate that much, as you'll be replacing that fat with lean muscle. What's important is that your overall health, your belt size, and appearance will change dramatically. So do not just say "I want to lose weight". Be specific and exact. Say "I will be 10% body fat", or 20% body fat, or whatever your goal is. Write it down.

2. What specifically will you give in order to become 10% body fat? Remember there is no such thing as something for nothing. Don't say, "I'll try to go to the gym 4 days a week". Say, "I go to the gym 4 days a week."

3. Pick an exact date when you will reach your burning goal. For example,"I am 10% body fat on April 15, 2016."

4. Follow a proven plan and start IMMEDIATELY whether you're ready or not. For example, follow a proven workout program like the monthly 4-week programs at our TeamLiveLean.com inner circle site. As a member, you will

also have access to our weekly cooking lesson recipe videos, meal plans, and grocery lists. I can't stress this enough. INVEST IN A PROVEN SYSTEM like TeamLiveLean. com. Not only do our workout and nutrition programs give you an exact step-by-step action plan, but by investing your hard earned money in yourself, you will also have extra motivation as you have more "skin in the game". Whether you're ready or not, go to TeamLiveLean.com right now, invest in yourself, and most importantly, put it into immediate action.

5. Take your answers from question 1-4 and write out a clear vision statement of what body fat % you will achieve, when you will accomplish it, what you will give in return to achieve it, and by following which specific plan. *"It's April 15, 2016 and I am 10% body fat. I go to the gym for 45-60 minutes, 4 days a week and follow the Team Live Lean workouts. I also love following the Team Live Lean meal plans. I follow the recipes and cook the delicious food in bulk every Sunday, and take the leftovers to work for lunches and snacks throughout the week. I love how I look, I love how I feel, I love my energy, and I love the Live Lean Lifestyle."*

6. Once you have it written out, read it out loud everyday when you first wake up and just before you go to bed. Find a quiet spot where it's just you and your thoughts. Claim this spot (and time) as your quiet zone. Make sure that when you read it, really feel like it's already happened and say it with emotion. Simply reading the words is not enough. You must believe! In the beginning you may feel silly and you may find it hard to visualize yourself already being that person, but if it's really what you desire, it will eventually come easy. Let your imagination go to work. This step is very important. Don't skip it!

7. Keep a written copy of your vision statement close by so you have access to it in the morning and night. Commit to memorizing it.

Great job. You have just defined your vision. Although it may seem overwhelming and look like Mount Everest right now, your stress and fear will disappear, once you break this vision down into smaller attainable goals. Don't worry, I'll show you how to do this in the upcoming chapters.

I hope you'll not only get a lot out of this exercise but it'll inspire you to take action. Re-read your Why and your vision twice a day, everyday to keep it top of mind.

ACTION STEP #3: WRITE DOWN YOUR GOALS

Now that I'm sure you've completed your Why and your vision, it's time to write down your goals. It has been proven that we are way more likely to achieve our goals when they are written down. This is because goals feel more real on paper compared to when they're just dancing around in your mind. Whenever you begin to deviate from your goal, refer back to your written goals.

Also since your vision may seem like it's a long way away, we're going to chunk it down into smaller and more achievable goals. It's like creating a roadmap to reaching your goal. Every small win brings you one step closer not only in the physical sense, but also the mental side. Before we chunk down your goal into smaller goals, we first must start with the end in mind. In other words, go back to what your ultimate goal is that you wrote down in your vision statement. Then we'll create the road map by breaking that big goal down into smaller achievable goals.

Chunking Down Your Goals:

If your goal is to lose 50 pounds of body fat, I want you to first focus on taking the first step. That means you have to lose 1 pound of body fat, then repeat that 49 more times. You start this journey by just finishing today's workout and eating one healthy meal at a time. I don't want you getting overwhelmed by the mountain of losing 50 pounds of fat in one year. Which focus point seems more stressful to you?

Completing one workout and losing 1 pound of fat or losing 50 pounds of fat? The answer is simple. Even though I know it's possible for a person to lose 50 pounds, the thought of it can even be overwhelming and stressful to me. But it's possible by taking it one step at a time. When you only focus on the big picture of what it will take to reach the mountain top, it's going to overwhelm you and make you not even want to start. Rather than trying to climb to the top of the mountain in one day, take it step-by-step. Break it down into monthly, weekly, and daily goals. Focus on one workout and one meal at a time. Losing 50 pounds of fat seems like a lot. But when you break it down over 52 weeks, that's only 1 pound per week. When you look at it that way, doesn't it seem much more obtainable?

Now it's time to show you how to break your burning goal down into smaller goals. It's time to create your Goal Mountain. On a piece of paper in your journal, draw a triangle (i.e. the mountain) with the peak at the top. The peak represents your main goal. Below your main goal are your monthly goals, below that are your weekly goals, and then below that are your daily goals. Each smaller short-term goal builds up to reach your main goal. This is your action plan at work.

Once you have filled in your Goal Mountain, keep a copy with you, post it around the house and review it first thing in the morning to stay focused for the day. Then before bed, journal how your day went, which goals you achieved, and what your action plan is tomorrow. Success breeds more success. Keep it positive. This will fuel your mind with thoughts of achievement towards achieving your goals while you sleep.

GOAL MOUNTAIN EXAMPLE:

John's goal is to be 10% body fat within one year. This will require John to lose 53 pounds of body fat in 52 weeks.

Here's how we figured that out. John's 5'11" and currently 230 pounds with a body fat of 30%. He currently has a decent amount of muscle since he plays recreational sports, but years of bad food decisions and lack of a consistent workout routine has created a thick layer of body fat over his muscle.

Based on a current body fat of 30%, John calculated his current body composition as 69 pounds of fat (230x0.30) and 161 pounds of lean body mass (230-69).

Lets work this out to calculate how much fat John will have to lose to create his ideal body fat %:

- Current lean body mass: 161 pounds
- Goal body fat%: 10%
- Goal weight: 177 pounds (161 x 1.10)
- Goal fat loss: 230 – 177 = 53 pounds of fat to lose

For John to hit his 10% body fat goal, he will have to lose approximately 53 pounds of body fat. This is an example of how to calculate and create a measurable fat loss goal.

MONTHLY GOALS:

Burn approximately 4.5 pounds of body fat per month (53 pounds/12 months)

WEEKLY GOALS:

Burn approximately 1 pound of body fat per week (4.5 pounds/4 weeks) via increased calorie burn and decreased calorie consumption:

Workout for 45-60 minutes, 5 days a week (creates increased calorie burn).

Consume 14,000 calories per week, thus creating a 3,500 calorie deficit at the end of the week (creates decreased calorie consumption).

DAILY GOALS:

Monday: Eat a good serving of protein, fat, and vegetables for breakfast. Bring leftovers from last night's dinner for a healthy lunch and snack at work. Prepare dinner in bulk to bring for lunch tomorrow. Log food in a journal to keep yourself accountable to your calorie goals. Bring your 1.5-liter water bottle to work so you can drink and refill it one time to ensure you're drinking at least 3 liters of water throughout the day. Enjoy your 45-60 minute circuit-training workout at 8pm.

Tuesday: Pretty similar to yesterday, eat a good breakfast, bring last night's dinner for lunch, and bring a bag of nuts and fruit for snacks along with protein powder in a shaker cup. Drink water. Go beast mode during your 45-60 minute workout at 8pm.

Wednesday: Eat according to your plan and drink water throughout the day. Make a list of healthy recipes to prepare in bulk for the second half of the week. Make a grocery list of items needed and pick them up at the store on your way home from work. Evening HIIT workout at the park at 8:00pm.

Thursday: You get the point…repeat.

Friday: Repeat.

Saturday: Enjoy a rest day from the gym but stay active by going for a long walk or play sports.

Sunday: Repeat with workouts, food, etc. but reflect on the past week. Celebrate your successful week by buying a new workout shirt or treat yourself to a massage. Always remember to celebrate your wins along your way up the Goal Mountain. Schedule your upcoming week. Prepare food in bulk for breakfast, lunch, dinners, and snacks. Go grocery shopping if needed.

Now it's your turn to create your very own Goal Mountain. Once you do, I promise you'll feel much more calm and focused. Although your goal may seem like a stretch now, by following these steps, you'll be feeling much closer than you think. Sure it's still a lot of work, but remember, there's no such thing as something for nothing. Enjoy the journey up your Goal Mountain and celebrate your little victories along the way.

Before moving on to the next chapter I just wanted to congratulate you on making it this far. By doing so, you're in the top 10% of people who buy an empowering book and actually read past the first chapter. So high-five to you for being persistent and taking action!

SECTION TWO
MASTERING YOUR THOUGHTS & WORDS

CHAPTER 2.1

BECOMING AWARE OF YOUR THOUGHTS & WORDS

You are a living magnet. What you attract into your life
is in harmony with your dominating thoughts.
- BRIAN TRACY

Science has proven it. Your thoughts are things. They can and will have a powerful impact on the outcome of your life. Your thinking can stop you from achieving your health, your career, and your relationship goals, or they can help you achieve excellence in all areas of life.

Whether positive or negative, your thoughts lead to creating the majority of your life experiences. And I say majority, because lets be real, horrible things, tragedies, and natural disasters happen to people. And of course no one "thinks" these horrible things into their life. But in most cases, the outcomes we experience in life are closely tied to the dominating thoughts we think every day.

It doesn't matter if it's building your dream body, landing the perfect job, or finding your soul mate. You can do it if you really desire it and you're willing to do anything, and risk everything, to achieve it.

Living Lean begins with the words you say and the thoughts you feed your mind every day. These nutrient-rich thoughts combined with a focused burning goal, an emotional why, a strong belief in your potential, an attitude of persistence, and of course my favorite, continuous daily action, will be your framework to acquiring the Live Lean Mindset.

If the thought of Living Lean excites you, but in your head you're dreading the thought of having to workout and eat healthy; take a deep breath and relax. Don't let this overwhelm you. The reason you feel stressed is because you're focusing on the wrong thing. As mentioned in the previous chapter, it can be completely overwhelming when we focus on all the things that need to be done at one time. That's why we completed the chunk it down exercise. Focus on completing one step, one workout, and one meal at a time.

Another big cause of feeling overwhelmed is that you're focusing on all the painful aspects of the process to Live Lean, rather than the positive outcomes they will create in your life. Stop filling your mind with stressful thoughts of all the "what I have to do's". Focus on the positive outcome of how you will feel after you complete the task. Let me ask you, have you ever heard anyone in the locker room after their workout say, "Man, I really wish I didn't come here to workout!". Probably not. Most people are on a natural high and filled with a sense of accomplishment after their workout.

This idea of focusing on the painful process happened to me plenty of times, especially when it came to writing this book. Writing a book seems like a colossal effort, and it is, but when I broke it down into smaller goals, chapter-by-chapter, page-by-page, and word-by-word, my stress decreased and my focus, energy, and desire increased. Whenever I got overwhelmed, I took a deep breath, and visualized how this book will be another tool to fuel my purpose of transforming the lives of 1,000,000 people via my Live Lean Transformation

Mission. Focus on the purpose of why you're doing it. I repeat, do not stress over all the tasks that need to be done at one time. As I showed you earlier, break your burning goal down into monthly, weekly, and daily goals. Then your Mount Everest will begin looking a lot more achievable as you progress.

If this still doesn't make sense, let me paint one more picture for you. Even though we all know exercising is important, it still amazes me that so few people make it a lifestyle habit. The number one excuse people always tell me is, "I don't have enough time." Is that really true? Be 100% honest with me. If I said to you, I'll give you one billion dollars if you lose 50 pounds, do you think you could find the time to exercise? I bet you could. Since nobody is going to give you a billion dollars, how does it sound if I told you exercise can create a life of happiness? That it can also give you massive amounts of energy to play with your kids. It can reignite your sex life with your significant other. It can make you feel young and sexy in your own skin. It can provide you with an unmatched sense of confidence in your abilities. I could continue but I think you get the point. Knowing that exercise can provide you with these outcomes, do you think you can now find the time? This is where you nod your head!

Without a doubt, you have the ability to change your health. You're just lacking the mindset to follow through. The real reason you're not making exercise a part of your lifestyle is because of the way you think about exercise. It's all about what you're focusing on. People who make exercise a part of their lifestyle are focusing on things that are very different than people who don't. Think about it, what thoughts and feelings come to your mind when I say exercise? You're probably thinking, this is going to be painful, uncomfortable, and a grueling experience. Your wish is my command. By associating exercise with pain and discomfort, you're creating the exact experiences that you're thinking. What you associate and focus on will determine if you are successful or not with making exercise a lifestyle habit. Focus on the positive outcomes of exercise, not the perceived pain.

Here is another quick example from my life. I remember when I was 13 years old. This was when I first thought about how amazing it would feel to go to the beach with friends and be able to confidently take my shirt off. Yes, I say confidently, because I feared those initial 10 seconds after I removed my shirt. Why? Well those initial 10 seconds make or break your confidence based on the looks from people, the comments, and the "harmless" jokes you receive.

To some of you, this may seem like a small thing, but at the time I struggled with self-confidence issues. I grew up 5 minutes from the beach, yet I can probably count on one hand how many times I went there with friends. It wasn't because I didn't have friends as I was actually a popular kid in school. But I struggled with how I felt about my body. I've been very open about my struggles on my Live Lean TV show. I remember countless hot summer afternoons that I'd skip out on the beach because I was uncomfortable being seen shirtless. At the time, I had skinny arms, a pudgy belly, and the pale skin color of an albino.

But here's the thing, although I looked decent in clothes, I think this illusion was one of the reasons that led to my self-confidence issues. Look at it this way, if you're a popular kid and you play sports, what happens when you feel like your body doesn't reflect those perceived characteristics. It's as if I felt like I was supposed to look a certain way to fulfill my role as the "popular athlete". This made me feel like a failure.

As time went on, I began to learn more about how my negative internal conversations with myself was making things worse. I became my own worst bully. Then one day when I was 23, I had a significant mindset shift. I decided that I had enough. I was no longer willing to accept living a life less than my potential. It was time to transform. Rather than allowing my low self-esteem to keep beating me up, I used my insecurities as fuel to create change. As you'll learn more about my story throughout this book, through the mentorship of various authors, I began my journey to master my thoughts and words. I began to implement various "self-talk" strategies to fill my mind with the positive nutrients I needed to take physical action. When I took consistent action, the results followed.

I remember when it all changed for me. I booked a tropical vacation with 10 of my closest friends to the Dominican Republic. This was my Live Lean "coming out" party. As soon as we walked off the plane, the hot Dominican sun gazed on my body. My first thought was, it's too hot to be wearing a shirt. Where as before, I'd probably sweat myself to death by keeping my shirt on to cover up my insecurities. I remember the feeling of actually looking forward to taking my shirt off. It was an eye opener for me. But first, we had to jump on a shuttle bus to take us to our resort. As soon as the bus dropped us off, I started to get nervous. But this time, I acknowledged the negative thoughts and quickly replaced them with positive thoughts. I was ready for this. My first real experience of taking my shirt off at the beach while feeling a sense of confidence was here. Without trying to make a scene, I quietly grabbed the collar of my shirt, pulled it over my head, and that's when it happened. This time, those initial 10 seconds were filled with looks of amazement and positive comments. Although there were still jokes, this time they were easier to take because they were making fun of the fact that I had a six pack and was ripped!

As I look back on those difficult times, I'm actually grateful to have experienced them. It pushed me to become a stronger person not only physically, but also helped me become more confident in my personal and professional career. It's now up to you to acknowledge where you are today and use this as your own fuel. This is your baseline. With persistent action on the steps discussed in this book, it's only going to get better from here.

CHAPTER 2.2

DEVELOPING A SUCCESS VS. FAILURE CONSCIOUS MINDSET

Success Trains. Failure Complains.
- UNKNOWN

If you've been following my Instagram, Facebook, and Twitter, you know I love sharing inspiring quotes. Reviewing motivational quotes first thing in the morning is a habit I've been following to help me set my intention for the day. Here's how my morning typically starts. I get up at 5am, hit the bathroom, pour a lemon water, then sit out on my deck and post a #LiveLeanMindset quote of the day to my social media channels. Based on these posts, many of my followers often ask me, *"Brad, what does it mean to have a Live Lean Mindset?"*.

To put it simply, a Live Lean Mindset is similar to a success conscious mindset. It's a strong belief in yourself that you have the ability to create your best life in all areas. So how do you acquire it? It's simple but not necessarily easy.

To shift your current mindset, it will take ongoing work. This work includes getting into the habit of continually creating re-affirming positive thoughts in your mind that lift you up to your highest possible potential. Your objective is to develop a mindset that will continuously drive you to take action towards achieving your goals no matter what obstacles get in your way (or what people may say). The evil brother of the success conscious mindset is the failure conscious mindset. This goes much deeper than the age old question, is the glass half empty or half full? It's about going after what you know you deserve and not accepting living a life of mediocrity.

I am still fascinated with the general idea that it's impossible for "average" people to get and maintain a flat stomach 365 days a year. If you think this, I'm calling you out right now. Using the word "impossible" is weak. It's used way too much in the ongoing conversations we have with ourselves and others. Sure, it's impossible to jump off the top of the Empire State Building, bare-naked, and land on your feet without injury. That's obvious. But how can people say it's impossible to get and maintain abs 365 days a year? I hear it all the time and I've always had a problem with that statement. The use of the word "impossible" limits your potential and keeps you in your comfort zone. We all have these types of people in our lives. They know all the reasons why things won't work and why things cannot be done. I classify these people as living with a failure conscious mindset.

On the other hand, people living with a success conscious mindset cut the word "impossible" out of their thoughts and vocabulary. They refer to it as, "I'm Possible". Success comes to people who think in abundance, they take personal responsibility for their outcomes, they're open, and they're truly ready to change. People with a failure conscious mindset think in poverty, they blame others for their current situation, and they're afraid to change. I see examples of this failure conscious mindset all the time on my Facebook Page. It's all negativity. They take zero responsibility for their actions and blame everything else for why things are not working for them. Don't be that person!

You may be saying, *"But Brad, I'm 300 pounds and I hate the way I look and feel."* Well first of all, think about it. Do you really think you're the only person that has ever been in this situation? Do you really believe there has never been another 300 pound person that has lost weight? I promise you, there are plenty of success stories from people just like you (just check out my Live Lean Success Stories page: www.LiveLeanTV.com/testimonials). The commonality amongst all these people is that they first changed their thoughts and words about being a victim, took responsibility for their past actions, and worked on developing a success conscious mindset. And don't worry, if you currently classify yourself as one of the many people having a failure conscious mindset, it's absolutely possible to change. That's what this book is all about.

Here's a real-life example of a person with a failure conscious mindset when it came to health. When I was 24, a friend of my parents made me a $20 bet that I'd have a beer belly by the age of 30. He thought it was impossible to maintain abs when you get older because everyone eventually gets a beer belly. His rationale, "that's just what happens to people when they age". Even though this guy was a former top tier athlete and a successful entrepreneur, his internal conversations and acceptance about aging and being out of shape took his health down the wrong path. This acceptance of his poor lifestyle habits created a life experience that created his outcome. This was a perfect example of adopting a failure conscious mindset and how your thoughts are things. In other words, if you believe something is impossible, it is. By the way, I never did collect on winning that $20 bet!

Compare that failure conscious mindset to this. Here's a real-world example from my life where my success conscious mindset created a positive outcome. When I first started my journey to Live Lean, I spent years following cookie cutter workouts and meal plans from fitness magazines. Even though

I worked hard, my results were minimal. I eventually became so confused at all the conflicting information, I almost gave up. That's when I decided to find just one person in the fitness industry that was getting the results I wanted. I eventually found this person, hired them, and followed their teachings. But here's where the "thoughts are things" mindset went to work not just for my body, but also for my career. I was amazed that my Los Angeles based coach was an entrepreneur who made a career out of becoming an online fitness "personality". He'd film his workouts and recipes, then post them online for people to watch. He set his own schedule, he worked to his own deadlines, and he was essentially the master of his own career. I was fascinated with this concept of living the entrepreneurial lifestyle.

At the time, I was working a full time corporate marketing job. As the years went by, I truly felt like I was not serving any purpose other than enticing people to drink more beer, buy more lottery tickets, and heat their homes with heating oil. Not my idea of fulfilling my life's purpose. I desired the same entrepreneurial lifestyle that my coach was living. And I'll be honest, before I began working on my mindset shift, I thought this entrepreneurial lifestyle was impossible for me to accomplish. After learning about the importance of mastering my thoughts, believing in myself, and taking massive action, my idea of "impossible" changed. As I was working towards building a success conscious mindset, I changed my attitude, I overcame my self-limiting beliefs, and I ultimately changed my life. But I didn't just sit on the couch thinking about the lifestyle I wanted. I fueled my thoughts with an emotional why and a strong purpose. I developed a never give up attitude of persistent action and created a burning desire to achieve my goal of living the entrepreneurial lifestyle. After a lot of struggle, hard work, and sleepless nights, I'm proud to say I'm now the master of my own career and truly living my purpose in life. My Live Lean Transformation Mission is currently educating, motivating and inspiring millions of men and women from over 180 countries.

However, I have to caution you. Changing a failure conscious mindset that may have been with you for years, will take time. So be patient. Creating a success conscious mindset is a continuous journey that will progressively get stronger every day you feed it. Think of it this way, every positive thought you think, just like every good workout or healthy meal, is like investing a dollar in your savings account everyday. It'll continue to compound and exponentially grow in value every single day. Keep nourishing your mind with success conscious thoughts. Every positive thought is a just another brick to build the essential foundation to Live Lean.

All of us are proving that it is possible to Live Lean 365 days a year. You can do it too without being a slave to the gym, without having to starve yourself of food, and without depriving yourself of a social life. It all starts with the mindset shift. High-five to you because you're now on your way to make that happen. Keep reading.

CHAPTER 2.3

CONTROLLING YOUR INTERNAL SELF-TALK

You are today where your thoughts have brought you;
you will be tomorrow where your thoughts take you.
- JAMES ALLEN

I remember the first time I walked over to the "big boy" dumbbell rack. That's the rack that holds all the dumbbells over 100 pounds. It was chest day, and according to the progression of my lifts, I was ready to move up from the 95-pound dumbbells to the big boys. Even though it was only a 5-pound increase, the thought of pressing 2 x 100-pound dumbbells over my face was way scarier than 2 x 95-pound dumbbells. As I approached the rack, my mind was filled with failure conscious thoughts such as, *"You're not strong enough to be at the big boy rack"* or *"How stupid will you look if you can't press them up"*. Regardless, I reached down, grabbed the dumbbells, carried them over to the bench, and attempted to lift them. FAIL. This was a classic failure conscious mindset example of failing first in the mind. In other words, before even physically trying, my mind was already made up that I couldn't lift the

100-pound dumbbells.

A week later, it was chest day again. And of course, my program had me set up to lift those damn 100-pound dumbbells again. But this time something was different. A few days before the workout I read an article on a topic called autosuggestion, or as I refer to it, self-talk. Essentially self-talk is a term that describes all the self-administered thoughts and feelings that reach our mind via our five senses: what we see, hear, taste, smell, and touch. For this example, I tapped into the hearing sense. I remember gripping the handles of the 100-pound dumbbells, looking straight into the mirror, and quietly mumbling to myself, "you can do this", "big chest", and "this is light weight". What happened next changed me. Even though the previous week I couldn't even lift them for 1 rep, this week I hoisted the weights up and proceeded to press them for 6 reps. Yes 6.

So what changed in 7 days? Did I get stronger? No. Did I take 4 scoops of pre-workout? No. I simply shifted my thoughts from a failure conscious mindset to a success conscious mindset. The words you say and the thoughts you think are powerful! That's the beauty of self-talk. Even if you've never heard of this word before, I have no doubt it's affecting your everyday life. Becoming aware of the communication between your conscious mind (where your initial thoughts take place) and your subconscious mind is critical. Those positive or negative thoughts will move from the conscious mind to the subconscious mind via repetitive self-talk. So be careful with what you are repeatedly thinking and saying to yourself.

As described in the dumbbell example above, this repetitive self-talk can work for you or against you. Fortunately, you have complete control over what reaches your subconscious mind and what is removed. But here's the key point. Having the *ability* to take control versus actually *taking* control are two separate things. Even though we have the ability to control this, most people don't which is a big reason why the world is filled with people living below their potential. A healthy outside, starts with a healthy inside. Anthony Robbins said it best when he said, "The quality of your life is the quality of your personal communications." Put simply, when we have an experience in life, you have the personal choice to either view it as good or bad. You have that inner communication with yourself. This ongoing self-talk will continually determine how you feel and act in the future.

For example, have you ever thought to yourself, "I hate training legs"? This is a classic example of negative self-talk. Simply put, the words you're saying or thinking are feeding your mind in a negative way. Here's the bad news. Ongoing negative self-talk will put a halt on all progress during your journey to Live Lean. Here's the good news. It can be reversed.

I remember I used to hate leg day. Nothing required more energy, more sweat, and created more muscle soreness than leg day. That's why I used to have really skinny legs and calves. I avoided training them because I associated negative feelings with them. I ended up being like most uneducated gym rats, where everyday was chest and bicep day. It's funny, because the reason I started working out was to build more self-confidence. But without knowing it at the time, what I was actually doing was hurting my self confidence by building a body that was out of proportion. My arms were big but my calves were skinny. In the beginning, I was the poster boy for one of those hilarious fitness *"Don't Skip Leg Day"* memes.

Fortunately, I took control of my self-talk and faced my fears. I now convinced myself to look forward to leg day. How did I transform from hating it, to loving it? Simple. Rather than seeing the pain, I envisioned the success of strong legs and well proportioned calves. I now train legs more than any other body part and have actually come to love leg days. I credit my dedication to leg training as one of the main reasons why my abs pop out 365 days a year. If you don't see how this is connected, you need to watch my YouTube channel, http://www.youtube.com/LiveLeanTV. Don't skip leg day no matter how big your legs currently are!

The point is, by associating positive outcomes that are created by a specific habit (even if you despise it in the beginning), you will eventually be able to transform negative thoughts into positive outcomes. Once again, rather than associating leg day with exhaustion and soreness, I shifted my mindset by associating it with getting leaner, getting abs, and getting more confidence.

Leg Day (old negative association) = exhaustion, soreness
Leg Day (new positive association) = improving my physique and overall confidence in life

This also works the other way around. I also associate negative habits like eating ice cream every day with negative outcomes like obesity, sickness, and lower self-esteem.

Ice Cream (old positive association) = tastes delicious, comforting
Ice Cream (new negative association) = fat, lazy, sick, and lower self-esteem

Creating these positive and negative associations with your thoughts can re-wire your brain and build long-term healthy habits.

For things to change for you, you have to change.
JIM ROHN

Throughout this book you're going to continually learn very simple strategies to help create more empowering self-talk communications. Key point, it doesn't take a complicated idea to change the way you think. It only takes an idea that you're willing to use. No matter what happens to you, it's not actually the "what happens" that makes the difference; it's what you decide to do with "the what happens". For things to change in your life for the better, YOU first have to change for the better.

You have to work on you, to develop a better version of you. If you think you've hit rock bottom, lets look at that as being a good thing. Why? Because since you're already at the bottom, there's only one way to go. Back to the top baby!

This section on self-talk is the corner stone of developing the Live Lean Mindset. If after reading this book you're still skeptical of self-talk, commit to reading this section out loud once every night until this belief is accomplished (I made it short for a reason). Just like the principle states, by repeatedly reading this section out loud, you will begin to believe. Commit to this, and you'll be well on your way to Living Lean.

CHAPTER 2.4

FEEDING YOUR SUBCONSCIOUS MIND

Whatever goal you give to your subconscious mind,
it will work night and day to achieve it.
- JACK CANFIELD

This is a big one. Over the past 10-20 years, the topic of the subconscious mind has been receiving a lot of mainstream media attention. The Merriam-Webster dictionary defines the subconscious mind as, *"existing in the part of the mind that a person is not aware of : existing in the mind but not consciously known or felt"*. To me that definition is a little vague. In an effort to ensure we're all on the same page, let me try and clearly articulate what the subconscious mind is in everyday human language.

We have a subconscious mind and conscious mind. The subconscious mind never takes time off. It's working and storing thoughts day and night. In other words, the subconscious mind is like a huge library with unlimited shelf space. Everything that happens to you in life is stored and retrieved as data in your mind library. Think of the subconscious mind as your garden. All the positive thoughts you repeatedly feed it represent beautiful flowers. But then come the weeds. These ugly creatures keep popping up based on the negative thoughts you repeatedly think. Like with everything, you are in control of your garden. Through repetitive self-talk, positive uplifting thoughts create more beautiful flowers. Repetitive negative self-defeating thoughts create those pesky weeds. When this gets out of control, they eventually take over and destroy your garden.

Your conscious mind has no memory. It's only dealing with and aware of the present moment. As Brian Tracy put it, *"Your conscious mind commands and your subconscious mind obeys".* I hope that explanation make more sense to you. If so, great. If not, don't worry about it. As you'll learn throughout this book, it's not about understanding how things work, it's more important to believe that it works and take action on it. I'll explain more of that later in the book. Lets keep moving on.

Success is not something you pursue. What you pursue will elude you. Success is something you attract and accumulate by the person you become.
- JIM ROHN

Nothing can be created until it is first formed as a thought. Your thoughts can act as magnets to attracting what you want, and what you don't want into your life. As we work on developing the Live Lean Mindset, it's super important to work on controlling your subconscious mind as much as possible. This is done by voluntarily feeding it with encouraging and positive emotional thoughts that are attached to your belief of achieving your goal. I'm referring to things you're passionate about such as your Why, your health goals, your belief in yourself, and your plan of action to achieve it. The more feeling or emotion you attach to your goals, the stronger the influence you will have over your subconscious mind. Unfortunately this works for both positive and negative emotions. In most cases the negative emotions will actually reach the subconscious mind much easier than the positive ones. This is why I keep mentioning how important it is to persistently practice positive emotional self-talk.

Emotion is the official language of the subconscious mind. Both positive and negative emotions cannot be held within the mind at the same time. Either one dominates at one time. It's essential that you realize this and take ownership of it. It's your role to keep your mind filled with positive thoughts. As always, practice and consistency will create this positive thinking habit. It will be challenging in the beginning, so strive for progress, not perfection.

With persistence, positivity will fill the storage space within your mind. It's your responsibility to block out all discouraging and negative thoughts that don't serve you in anyway. It'll either support or disrupt your Live Lean journey depending on how you train it. The thoughts you feed your mind is no different than the food you feed your body. Think of positive thoughts as a healthy meal comprised of a grass fed filet mignon, an organic salad, and a big glass of water. This meal is full of nutrients to help you be strong and healthy. Think of negative thoughts as potato chips, cookies, and crackers. These foods are not only void of any nutrients, but they'll also pull nutrients away from your body. Your subconscious mind won't remain idle. It's always being fed either positive or negative thoughts. It's on you to be aware and control which one you want to fuel your mind with.

I say be aware, because without even knowing it, you're bombarded every minute with all sorts of negative (and some positive) stimuli that is reaching your subconscious mind. It's your job to be the gatekeeper. You can do this by shutting off the stream of negative energy by turning off the news, stop reading gossip magazines and blogs, and limit contact with energy zapping negative people.

You'll know it when you feel it. Think about it, how do you feel after watching the news about war, murder, famine, and crime? Probably not very positive. Compare that with reading an uplifting book, watching a Ted Talks presentation on NetFlix, finishing a sweaty workout, or simply going for a walk with a loved one (your dog included). One fuels the mind and body with positive thoughts and energy, while the other depletes us of energy.

I repeat, you need to be like a big and strong nightclub bouncer to your mind. Protect it by limiting all undesirable thoughts. But don't stress over it. Just become aware of it. We're not trying to be perfect. We're just trying to improve our life. Take this one day at a time. Don't expect to change your life in one day.

Here's an example from my life that I've never shared with you before. Back in 2006, before finding my passion in health and fitness, I started investing in real estate. Yes, I wanted to become the next Donald Trump. At the time, I really thought real estate investing was my passion. I was hooked on watching those flipping shows on TV, and became convinced that real estate would be the key to unlock my financial freedom. I read a ton of books, I attended seminars, and eventually hired a team to find me undervalued properties that I could purchase, renovate, and rent out to tenants. Within 6 months, I had closed deals on two apartment buildings. I was young and naive, had no clue what I was doing, and scared out of my mind. Once the deals closed, I thought the hard work was done. Boy was I wrong. Next up was setting budgets and finding, negotiating, and hiring contractors to renovate the units. Once I hired someone, I remember thinking, what a pain in the butt, but so glad I'm finally past the hard part. Then came all the headaches of budget overtures, finding disasters behind the walls, water pipe breaks, flooding, and I could go on and on. I eventually got passed all that, and took a huge sigh of relief when the renovations were done (or so I thought). Then I moved on to the "easy" part, finding good qualified renters. After all I've been through getting up to this point, I assumed the worst was behind me. So wrong. My tenants and the buildings became my worst nightmare. I remember being so negative about the whole experience. I hated it. Every time my phone rang or every time I opened my email, I would literally get a pit in my stomach thinking it was a tenant or an issue with the building. Disaster after disaster was happening. Late night parties, domestic violence, drug dealers, missed rent payments, more required renovations, etc.

At the time I was a ball of negative stress. Without knowing it, I kept filling my subconscious mind with negative thoughts. My negative thinking was on auto-pilot. For example, whenever it rained out, my thoughts instantly when straight to worrying about the roof leaking. Whenever it was cold out I kept worrying about the water pipes freezing and breaking. I would go to bed with bad thoughts, which led to having nightmares about those thoughts, and then I'd wake up in the morning, and yes, I'd have an email that those things actually happened overnight. I'm 100% serious.

At this point I knew I had to change. I'll say it right now, if I die before I'm 100 years old, I would blame it on that time of stress. However, like I said earlier, I used these negative experiences to take action and grow. This is when I started reading more about the subconscious mind. I learned I could change my mental impulses by feeding my mind with positive thoughts of my desired outcomes. I even started meditating and repeating positive affirmations to myself. Look at it this way. Remember the last time you told a white lie at work to cover up missing a deadline? At the time you told the lie, of course you didn't believe it because it wasn't true. However, since you had to keep telling more and more people the lie to cover your back, eventually you actually begin to believe it yourself. That is the power of making repeated affirmations. Eventually your subconscious picks up on it, accepts it as reality, and soon becomes a belief. Get it?

Now the key is to use affirmations to create positive beliefs, not lies! A positive example is when your beliefs lead you to take massive action towards achieving your goal. Here's an example of a positive affirmation I began implementing. Anytime a negative thought about a bounced rent check came into my thoughts, I immediately acknowledged it, and replaced it with the following affirmation:

"I am a successful real estate investor, with happy and respectful tenants who pay their rent on time."

Any time I heard the phone ring and the negative thoughts began to form in my head, I immediately acknowledged it, and replaced it with that positive affirmation. Even though I still received the occasional issue, things did eventually improve over time. Do not become discouraged if nothing changes for you immediately. Consistency eventually creates habit. And with habit comes change. Trust the process and be patient. I can't explain it any other way, other than saying this practice made me feel better, I was less stressed, and I wasn't so negative all the time.

You may be wondering if I still own these properties. The answer is no. Back in 2011, I eventually sold these properties, for a profit, and found my real, life-long passion in helping people Live Lean. Like all things Live Lean related, the concept behind my mindset shift was simple, but it wasn't easy. It will be challenging and will require a lot of willpower in the beginning. But just like detoxing your body of sugar, it is hard in the beginning, but you eventually adapt and eating healthy becomes a habit. Your mind will follow suit as you become more persistent with creating these new thinking habits. No one else can do it for you. It's on you.

Once again, I know it may not make sense or may seem too "woo woo", but I encourage you to remain open to this concept. Try to accept the reality that the thoughts you feed your subconscious mind will either take you closer to or further away from your goals of Living Lean.

And when I say your "goal of Living Lean", this can mean different things to different people. It's your responsibility to be clear on what Living Lean means to you. As I shared earlier, in the beginning of my personal journey, Living Lean meant feeling the confidence to be comfortable enough to take my shirt off in front of other people, and maintain that feeling 365 days a year. This is important. Anyone can get in shape, but it's the people who have acquired the Live Lean Mindset that can maintain their health 365 days a year. I do not believe in "dieting" or "cardio-ing" yourself to death before a last minute beach vacation. People Living Lean are healthy and maintain their lean physique all year round. Like it did for me, eventually this new sense of physical confidence will transfer over into other areas of confidence in your life. When you're able to transform your body, you're able to transform your business, your personal relationships, and your finances.

So take some time if you haven't already done so and clearly articulate what Living Lean means to you. Write it down and be persistent in achieving it. I hope this is starting to make sense to you. This is why we should be writing out our goals and repeating them out loud as if you're already in possession of them. By repeatedly reading it out loud with a true feeling of emotion and belief of it happening, you're feeding your subconscious mind with thoughts of having already accomplished your goal.

However simply reading the words is not enough. It's critical that you read them with emotion and belief. It has been shown that your subconscious mind will only act upon repetitive thoughts that are mixed with feeling. This lack of emotion and belief is one of the reasons why so many people don't see results when implementing self-talk techniques. They just don't believe in the words they are saying. And I get it, at first you may feel awkward with talking to yourself out loud. If so, don't give up. Remember, persistence is key in making self-talk work for you. Eventually it will come to you. But as I said earlier in this book, there's no such thing as something for nothing. You must work for it. You must commit to taking action and remain persistent with feeding your garden (your subconscious mind) with flowers (positive thoughts). If you tried but are not seeing results, I want you to concentrate harder, and try more. When I say concentrate, I mean when you close your eyes, you should visually see the exact physical appearance of the person you will become. If your burning goal is to be 10% body fat, you need to concentrate so hard, that you can see and feel yourself at 10% body fat. I want you to feel yourself running around with your kids on a hot summer day. Concentrate on the warm air, the sounds of your kids laughing, the feeling of happiness you have to be able to keep up with your kids. This is the type of concentration you should have when you're feeding your mind. You must believe it! I must keep repeating this because it's critical in order for your subconscious mind to pick up and act on it.

In addition to visualizing yourself as already having the body you want, you must also see yourself putting in the work and taking the necessary action to achieve your body. You can't just sit on the couch thinking about it. Action is required. If you're planning on going to the gym the next morning, before you go to sleep, I want your final thoughts to be visualizing yourself waking up and going to the gym. I want you to feel the sweat and feel the muscle burn caused by lifting weights. Visualize yourself going to the grocery store, buying healthy foods, having fun cooking, and eating those foods for breakfast, snacks, lunch, and dinner.

Bottom line. Never give up. Trust the process. If you really want this, you can do it. Focus on it as if it's a habit. Habits create action. When this happens, your subconscious mind will work in your favor. In the coming chapters I'm going to share another personal story about a business proposal that came out of no where that essentially saved my career. If this business proposal didn't come when it did, who knows what I'd be doing right now. Once again, trust the process!

If you're still skeptical, do me a favor and make the commitment right now just to be open to the possibility. Once you commit to it, the awkward feelings will eventually go away. Talk to yourself with a strong sense of belief. Feel it already being in your possession. Eventually this will become second nature, you will begin to gain control over your subconscious mind, and things will mysteriously begin to happen. I personally have so many examples of this happening to me in the last 3 years (attracting a beauty named Ms. Jessica Rumbaugh being the most important one).

CHAPTER 2.5

VISUALIZING AND IMAGINING YOUR SUCCESS

If having others believing in you and your dream was a requirement for success, most of us would never accomplish anything.

- JACK CANFIELD

Lets have some fun with this chapter. It's creative, it's imaginative, and it's going to make you feel young, wild, and free. It's time to start living the life you've imagined. Your Live Lean transformation may seem far away now. But what's going to keep you committed, through all the ups and downs, is your burning desire to reach your goal. If your desire is intense, you should have no problem visualizing and imagining yourself achieving it. I want you to become so determined, so committed, and so fired up, that you can close your eyes and already see it. Saturate your mind with feelings of having already obtained your goal every night before you go to bed. It's important to understand that every successful person in life who has overcome significant challenges, or experienced greatness, has first started their journey with a dream. If you cannot see it in your imagination, you will have a hard time seeing it come to life. Imagination and visualization is one of the main practices that allows your subconscious mind to receive ideas, plans, and your vision for your ideal life.

Let me ask you, when you were a kid, what did you want to be when you grew up? I wanted to be a fire truck, not a fireman, but a fire truck. True story. As kids, we let our imagination run wild. Then we become adults and the shackles of what we once wanted out of life, ties us down. It's time to remove those shackles on your imagination and remember what it was like to be a kid again. This chapter is all about formulating and devising the idea in your mind about what you want your health to look like. Living Lean, like most breakthroughs, starts first with an idea. Have fun with it. It's time to paint the picture in your mind what a life of Living Lean looks and feels like. Maybe it's being full of energy and running around with your grandkids. Maybe it's walking down the beach full of confidence in your favorite swimsuit. Regardless of what it is, it's time to imagine everything you want in life as vividly and real as possible. How do you do this? Lets get started.

I remember when I was 29 years old. Most people would be envious of the position and the life I was living. However, I imagined something different. For some reason I wasn't happy with my current situation. I was employed with an up and coming company, I was making a decent paycheck, and I was married to a beautiful and successful woman. I was this…I was that…but now that I look back on it, I wasn't happy. I imagined something different for my life. I imagined living in a different part of the world. I imagined having the freedom to make a living by pursuing my passion. I imagined having the ability to inspire people all over the world to live a healthier lifestyle. I simply imagined a different life than the one I was currently living. I can't say for sure if this imagined life led to the breakup of my marriage or the loss of my childhood friendships. But I can say I feel like the life I was imagining was taking me in a different direction. Although I'm still on the journey towards living the life I imagined back in 2009, I can say I'm much closer today than I was 6 years ago.

The same can be said about my fitness journey. My imagination was stimulated by my burning desire to achieve a body image that I was confident and proud of. It's often said, yet often ignored that we can create anything we can imagine. The most successful entrepreneurs, musicians, and entertainers all had a powerful and creative imagination. For example, back in the 1980's, Bill Gates said he imagined that every home in America would have a computer. It was a crazy idea at the time, but thinking about it now, it's actually crazy to think of a home without a computer. Ideas are products of the imagination. Imagination, like belief, plays a huge role when it comes to achieving your Live Lean goals.

Now let me ask you, do you feel like you lack a creative imagination? If so, I have to challenge you on your burning desire. Is it really something that your strongly want to achieve? If so, commit right now to developing and using your imagination to help achieve your burning desire to Live Lean. Your imagination is just like a muscle. When it's not put to work, it becomes weak and inactive. So put it to work! Think about your imagination as your wingman when it comes to growing a strong belief in yourself. Creating a strong, active, and vivid imagination is just another piece of the overall formula to Live Lean. It's main role is to help visualize, mold, and shape the required belief you must have in your abilities to achieve your burning desire.

After you finish reading this book, make a note in your journal to come back to this chapter so you don't forget to put your imagination to work. Remember, if you can't imagine and visualize yourself there, how do you think you're going to get there?

IMAGINE THAT YOU CAN AND WILL DO IT!
SEE YOURSELF IN POSSESSION OF IT.
IMAGINE THAT YOU ENJOY TAKING ACTION
TOWARDS IT EVERYDAY!

It's worked for me and it's worked for others. Imagine your life before you go to bed. Imagine your life before you get up in the morning. Become consumed with this burning desire and always remember, the only limitation you will face is the limitation that you created in your mind. Where there's a will, there's a way. Imitate the lifestyle, the habits, and the actions of the people that you admire and are getting the results you want for your life. I always laugh when people tweet me saying, *"Before putting anything in my grocery cart, I always ask myself, 'would Brad put this in his cart?'".* Reshape your life, your choices, and your decisions by feeling, taking action, and emulating your mentors.

Pretend like I'm walking down that grocery aisle with you. If I was, would you really put those cookies in your cart? Pretend like Jessica and I are coming over for dinner. Would you really serve that frozen meal? Visualize me working out beside you at the gym. If I was, would you really only lift those 10 pound dumbbells or would pick up the intensity? Would you squeeze out one more burpee? Could you add another few pounds to the bar? You have become the person you are today based on the dominating thoughts you think, the daily choices you make, and the desires you have. How would all of that change, if I was right beside you every waking hour of the day? How would your decisions change? How would your choices differ? How would your actions line up with your goals? You can apply this imagination principle to any area of your life that you want to improve. Find a person who you admire and has the particular characteristics and results that you want to acquire. If you want to get control of your financial life, imagine Warren Buffet at your side. Would he approve of your choices? Or if you want to improve your career, imagine Tony

Robbins sitting at your office desk. Would you be doing the things you're currently doing if you knew Tony Robbins was watching you?

Imagination is everything. It is the preview of life's coming attractions.
- ALBERT EINSTEIN

Let your imagination run wild here guys. Act as if. It's not creepy. It's not weird. Imagination is a tool to help you get what you want out of life. Be open to it. Although strengthening your imagination may seem like a slow process in the beginning, with consistent practice (like everything), it will be another amazing tool in your Live Lean toolbox. If you can't quite visualize it yet, do not give up. Give yourself permission to dream again just like when you were 5 years old. Spend more time dreaming about your life, rather than watching other people live their life on TV. Spend at least 5 minutes a day, with your eyes closed visualizing the new you. Trust me, this is the easy and fun part of the process. But remember, dreams without action do not become reality, they're called fantasies.

I once dreamed of achieving a body where I'd be confident in taking my shirt off. I dreamed of a career where I'd help inspire millions of people to build more confidence and achieve a life of health. I mixed that dream, with an action plan, a commitment, and a burning goal to succeed no matter what. That's the Live Lean mindset you need to not just accomplish your health goals, but more importantly create a healthy lifestyle that allows you to maintain them forever.

Everything you think, say, and do needs to be intentional and aligned with your purpose, your values, and your goals.
- JACK CANFIELD

So far we've learned that thoughts are things. The thoughts and self-talk you have with yourself every day will either have a positive or negative affect on the outcome of your life. It's up to you right now, to get your mind right, to get your thoughts working in your favor, and stay committed to never giving up on your journey to Live Lean. Your thoughts truly matter. Read that sentence again, and again, and again. That statement is one of the most important steps that I need you to stamp in your mind. Once you acquire this new way of thinking, it will become one of your greatest assets in all areas of life. Having the knowledge to turn your thoughts into real life positive experiences is a game changer. Even if you're starting from zero like I did, knowing what you want, and having the initiative, belief, and ultimately the commitment to overcome obstacles no matter what, is key to achieving your goals.

The personal experiences I've shared with you in this section have changed my thinking forever. I've learned to overcome and embrace failures as they always teach us lessons. It's up to you to find those lessons and learn from them. You can have a life of poverty, a life of low energy, a life of pain, or you can choose to have a life of Living Lean. The power to control your thoughts, either positively or negatively, is within you.

Thank you for keeping an open mind as we continue our Think And Live Lean journey together. In the next chapter, I'm going to share one of the most important steps as well as more personal experiences of how I made it happen in my life.

LIVE LEAN ACTION STEPS

Here are 2 action steps to begin mastering your mind and creating a Live Lean Mindset of success.

ACTION STEP #1: AFFIRMATIONS

First step is to get into the habit of immediately replacing negative thoughts and self-talk with healthier, positive affirmations.

For example, every time you say to yourself: *"I'm going to skip today's workout because I'm feeling tired and lazy"*, immediately identify that it's a negative thought, and correct it by following up with a positive affirmation such as: "I'm going to go to the gym right now because I love the rush of endorphins and energy I get from finishing an awesome workout."

Now I want you to make a list of the top 5 negative thoughts that continue to invade your mind.

YOUR TOP 5 NEGATIVE THOUGHTS

1.
2.
3.
4.
5.

Great job. Before I get you to write out your positive affirmations, here are two simple tips I want you to follow:

1. **Only use positive words.** When you use a negative word within a positive phrase, it has been proven that your subconscious mind will continue to focus on that negative word. For example, don't say "I will go to the gym so I don't feel tired and lazy anymore". Even though it's somewhat of a positive phrase, your mind will still hear and focus on the negative words being used: tired and lazy. A better positive affirmation is like the one I wrote earlier: *"I am going to go to the gym right now because I love the rush of endorphins and energy I get from finishing an awesome*

workout." See the difference? I used positive words such as "endorphins" and "energy" rather than negative words such as "lazy" and tired".

2. **Only use present tense.** Using present tense places more focus on the now as opposed to having to accomplish something in the future. For example, rather than saying *"I will go to the gym…"* say *"I am going to the gym…"* May seem silly but your subconscious mind sees it as happening now versus something happening at an unknown time in the future.

Using these two simple tips, I now want you to write 5 positive affirmations to use to immediately replace those 5 negative thoughts you listed above.

YOUR TOP 5 POSITIVE AFFIRMATIONS

1.
2.
3.
4.
5.

Don't be shy. You can do this. No one else needs to see this so make sure you're coming from a place of honesty. You can use these affirmations in any area of your life; it doesn't just have to be about your health. For example, here are 5 affirmations that I use for my career:

Brad's Top 5 Negative Thoughts

1. I don't have the "It Factor" to become a mainstream spokesperson in the fitness industry.
2. There's not a big demand for this type of book from me.
3. My YouTube channel and social media channels will always just have a medium sized following.
4. Why take the risk of investing more money into my business (and possibly not getting any return) when I'm comfortable where I currently am.

5. That brand won't want me as a spokesperson for their company.

Brad's Top 5 Positive Affirmations

1. I have all the tools to be a mainstream spokesperson in the fitness industry. I'm living the lean lifestyle, I have the knowledge, I have the look, I have the charisma and personality, and I've proven that I can connect with people and create positive changes in their lives.

2. This book has changed the lives of many people and is a top seller in my portfolio of products.

3. My YouTube channel and social media channels continue to reach more people and grow larger every day.

4. Investing in my business (and ultimately myself) always gives me positive returns.

5. I bring instant credibility and value to every brand I represent.

See that wasn't so hard. Once you're finished writing your affirmations, lets move on to the last action step of this chapter.

ACTION STEP #2: THINGS YOU LOVE ABOUT YOURSELF

It's time to show yourself some love and create an inventory list of all the things you love about yourself. This should be an ongoing list that you keep updating in your journal. Do I sense some hesitancy on your part to complete this action step? Don't be scuuuuured.

Creating a list like this is not arrogant or shallow. Once again, it's meant to help you highlight all the positive things about you as a person. I'm sure you can list at least 5 things, right?

Okay, how about I break the ice by telling you 5 things I love about myself:

Brad's 5 Things He Loves About Himself

1. I love my continuous and never ending commitment to self-improvement.
2. I love my smile.
3. I love my creativity in the kitchen and my ability to make a delicious meal out of any mixture of healthy ingredients.
4. I love my physique.
5. I love that I've transformed myself from being a shy and risk-adverse person into someone that has the guts to push myself out of my comfort zone and continue to go after and create the life I deserve.

I could go on and on, but I'll stop because it's now your turn. Write down your list. Then whenever you're having a bad day, come back to this list for re-assurance that you my friend, are indeed freaking awesome.

By implementing these action steps, you will not master your mind overnight. It's a continuos journey. But trust me, when you commit to replacing your negative self-talk with positive affirmations, as well as keeping an ongoing list of why you're awesome, day by day you will be making positive steps towards mastering your thoughts.

Once again, every positive thought is another deposit straight into your Live Lean Mindset piggy bank. The more positive deposits you make, the more habits you'll be forming, and the compounding will grow exponentially.

ACTION STEP#3: VISUALIZE YOURSELF AS THE PERSON YOU WILL BECOME

Start scheduling in at least 5 minutes a day to visualize yourself as the person you will become. Pick a time and stick to it. Maybe it's as soon as you get up, or maybe you prefer just before bed. Sit quietly. Close your eyes. Take deep breaths. See and feel yourself as the person you want to become. Feel yourself with more energy, feel how strong your new self is, feel your clothes fitting you better. Keep filling your mind with thoughts of who you will become.

If you've never visualized before, you will feel weird in the beginning. Your mind will wander, you'll have problems focusing, but trust the process (it's just 5 minutes a day). Eventually your mind will quiet down, you will feel a sense of peace, and you'll actually look forward to these 5 minutes. After 5 minutes becomes easy, simply add another minute every week and work your way up to 20 minutes.

Promise me that you won't skip out on this. Creating a new you requires new habits. Plan in this 5 minutes just like it's a doctor's appointment that you would not miss. Enjoy the gainz!

SECTION THREE
AWAKENING YOUR POWER OF BELIEF

CHAPTER 3.1

BUILDING A STRONG BELIEF IN YOURSELF

The number one problem that keeps people from winning in the United States today is lack of belief in themselves.
- ARTHUR L. WILLIAMS

Your beliefs lead to your behaviors. Your behaviors lead to your results. So the question is, do you believe in yourself? Think about it. Do you really believe you can accomplish your burning desire to Live Lean? Understanding that you are in complete control of your destiny is absolutely critical to accomplishing your goal. Having a strong belief in yourself will positively change the ongoing thoughts and outcomes created by your mind. You can think all the positive thoughts you want, but without truly believing it, you won't be enticed to take the necessary action. Let me state this clearly and concisely because it's so important. Positive thoughts are pointless if you don't believe you have the ability to achieve them. Why? It's a simple formula.

No Belief In Yourself = No Action = No Results

Read that statement as many times as you can until it sinks in. Belief in yourself is essential to all your goals, including Living Lean. Belief is the reason why miracles happen. How many times have you heard of people who have been diagnosed by doctors to never walk again, then end up leaving the hospital on two feet.

Belief is the main reason why I never gave up on my online fitness business. Even when I was working 16 hour days, 7 days a week and making less than $2,000 a year from online sales, I believed I could do it. These miracles happen every day to people with a strong belief in something. Listen to any athlete after winning a big game. They either credit their success to a strong belief in their abilities or a strong belief in a higher power that is looking out for their best interests. I'd be willing to bet one of the issues holding you back is your lack of belief in yourself or something greater.

> *Don't wish things were easier, wish you were better.*
> *- JIM ROHN*

Is it possible after all those years of self-defeating beliefs to finally start believing in yourself today? Absolutely. Will it be easy? No. I'll say it again. Anything worthwhile in life, takes persistent work. Since you've come this far in the book, I take it that you're committed to the ongoing required work. But before we get to the techniques to change your limiting beliefs, let me first share another personal example from my life.

I share these examples to prove to you that I've personally hit many lows in my life. In other words, I get where you're coming from. Life is tough and will continue to challenge your belief in your abilities every day. I remember when I first graduated from university with a degree in business and a major in marketing. Since I had my golden ticket, I thought it was going to be easy to land my dream job on Madison Avenue. Boy was I wrong. I sent out resume after resume with no success. Not even a job interview. At this point I remember second guessing my abilities, my self-worth, and my overall purpose. As I mentioned earlier in the book, I ended up taking many jobs that I absolutely despised.

You have to understand, while growing up I loved my jobs. Entering the workforce at the age of 16, I loved working at a golf course. I then went on to work at an awesome sporting goods store. During my studies, I even landed three internships working in the corporate world. In other words, I was very fortunate growing up to always land a pretty cool job. Not that there's anything wrong with it, but I was always grateful to never have had to sling fast food burgers and french fries.

So after graduating with a degree, it was a real shock to my confidence that the only jobs I could get were cutting grass and working in a wood factory. These negative thoughts and beliefs about my abilities quickly transferred to my subconscious mind. Just another example of how are thoughts are things. I still remember having vivid nightmares about being sent back to grade one in school. But in my dreams I wasn't a 6 year old kid like the rest of the kids in grade one. I was a 23-year-old adult. I became so sensitive about my lack of employment, one night I physically attacked one of my best friends who was poking fun at me. If you know me personally, you'd know I don't have one violent bone in my body. However at that point in my life, my confidence and belief in myself was at an all time low. I was hurting and I just lost it.

Eventually through hard work, determination, and the help of the steps discussed in this chapter, I was able to overcome my lack of belief in myself and my abilities. But it didn't just all of a sudden happen on one exact day. As always, it's a process that occurs over time. Fast forward 10 years, and here I am on the journey towards living my dream life. Everything started changing when I changed my mindset. In particular, a mindset based on a belief that I have everything inside of me to control my destiny. I am no different than you. Our brains are both wired the same way.

> *Your brain is designed to solve any problem and reach any goal that you give it.*
> *- JACK CANFIELD*

Over the years, I've become fascinated with the human brain. It's one thing to have your body performing at optimal levels, but just imagine what you could achieve in your life if you unleashed the true power of your brain.

Ever since I saw the movie "Limitless" with Bradley Cooper, I've always wondered how different my life would be if I had the ability to use 100% of my brain. In the movie, he takes a super drug called "NZT" which allows him to tap into his full potential. However like most powerful drugs, taking NZT came with severe withdrawal and premature death. That's not how we roll.

So how can you optimize your brain to create the healthiest, most successful, and confident version of yourself? Well first of all let me be clear. I am not a neurologist. Throughout my journey, I have simply become more aware that our brain is more powerful than we give it credit for. In my readings, I've learned scientists are discovering that there are up to 14,000,000,000 nerve cells in the cerebral cortex. With that said, it's hard to believe the human brain is only capable of performing physical functions of the body. More and more studies are coming out that show our inner self is more connected to other external forces than most of us are aware of or open to exploring.

I do not claim to be an expert in this, nor do I have a true understanding of why it works. But then again, I'm also ignorant to the inner workings of how electricity, gravity, thunder and lightning, or even why the internet works. But I know when I flip on a light switch, the room will light up. I know if I step off the edge of a cliff I will fall, and I'll find a search engine if I type "Google" into a web browser. It just works.

So why would I limit my belief regarding the power of our brains just because I don't physically see it or truly understand the force behind it? I simply choose to remain open and believe what many scientists are proving to be real. Even though I'm still on my journey in many aspects of my life, I have practiced the steps covered in this book for over 7 years. I'm amazed at the things that are happening in my life today because of what I thought, imagined, and believed over the past 7 years.

CHAPTER 3.2

KEEPING TRACK OF YOUR LIFE WINS

You have to believe in yourself when no one else does.
That's what makes you a winner.
- *VENUS WILLIAMS*

So far we've discussed how believing in yourself and your abilities is a critical step to creating a Live Lean Mindset. I'd be willing to bet a vast majority of you reading this book will struggle with the concept of believing in yourself. It's sad but it's true. Life may have beaten you down so much that your belief in your abilities is next to zero. I wish I had a quick belief pill to prescribe to you but there are no such short cuts. The best technique that worked for me to increase my belief in myself was keeping a running list of my "Life Wins". This is one of my favorite tools to go back to when life's playing hardball with me. I keep an ongoing list outlining all my life wins in my journal. These wins can be big wins like getting a promotion at work, as well as little wins like going to the gym even when you didn't feel like it at the time.

Each entry in this list is more proof that your life is filled with successes. Unfortunately, for whatever reason, we always tend to focus more on the failures. This quickly cripples our belief in our abilities to accomplish big things in life. This is why it's so important to make contributions to your Life Wins list. You have to re-program your mind to focus more time on the wins and less time on the failures.

It's hard to describe the feeling I get every time I review my Life Wins list. I often forget all of the accomplishments that I've achieved so far in my life. Reviewing this list is like a shot of adrenaline. The world becomes your playground. Your goals become more achievable because of everything you've overcome and accomplished in the past. You ultimately begin to believe in yourself. Here's an example of a few of the items from my Life Wins list. This is an ongoing list that I continue to add to.

Brad's Life Wins List

1. Paid my way through University and graduated debt free
2. Started my own full-time fitness business
3. Became certified in fitness, nutrition, and wellness
4. Published a book
5. Filmed a DVD workout program
6. Moved to Los Angeles
7. Married a women who shares the same vision and values as I do
8. Paid to speak on stages in front of thousands of people
9. Paid fitness model (including a cover of a magazine)
10. Named "1 of America's Hottest Personal Trainers"

Once you create this mindset of belief, your new positive thoughts backed by strong emotions, along with persistent action will turn your burning desires into reality. On the contrary, negative beliefs and negative feelings breed more poverty. Once you begin to truly believe that you are in control and are the creator of your future, then and only then are you open to obtaining your goal of Living Lean.

When you create your Life's Wins at the end of this chapter, remember to write them and say them in a positive and uplifting way. It's time to pat yourself on the back.

> *There are no limitations to the mind except those we*
> *acknowledge.*
> *- NAPOLEON HILL*

Always remember this key point: your mind becomes influenced most by the thoughts that dominate it. Choose to dominate it with self-empowering thoughts and protect it from all negative, self-limiting emotions and thoughts. A mind dominated by positive thoughts creates a belief in oneself and one's abilities.

As I've said countless times. I continue to work on building my confidence everyday. Now don't get me wrong, I've come a long way since my days as an awkward and shy kid. One of the greatest feelings I had was when my brother, one of the people I'm closest with and respect so much, commented on how much I've grown.

CHAPTER 3.3

OVERCOMING YOUR FEARS

Fear is what stops you…courage is what keeps you going.
- *UNKNOWN*

Everything that has been created in life was first born as a thought. With that said, fear can be controlled and mastered since fear is just a state of mind. Nothing more, nothing less. However, to shift your current mindset, you first have to be open to the fact that change is inevitable. Many times people think they want to transform their body, but they do not realize that to permanently change, you must first change your mindset. The new shift in thinking must prepare the mind to receive and apply new daily actions that will eventually turn into life-long habits. It requires you to get a better understanding of the things that are currently getting in the way and stopping you from accomplishing your desires. Napoleon Hill broke it down into three complementary buckets.

Indecision, doubt, and fear.

I say "complementary" because one typically feeds

into another. Think about it. People often lack ambition and for some reason have a willingness to accept their poor health. Call it laziness, lack of initiative, lack of discipline, or zero self-control. They're essentially indifferent about their health. They take it for granted and consider it normal to have no energy and a flabby belly. This indecision usually creates doubts or excuses why they can't do it or why they continuously fail to get in shape when they do try. To make themselves feel better, they find fault and criticize other people who are Living Lean by saying they have no fun in life and need to live a little. They continuously look at the negative side of Living Lean. Thinking only of the things they'll have to give up, the pain, and the agony of weight loss. They focus on the pain points rather than concentrating on the way they'll feel once they reach their goals. They're always waiting for the perfect time to start which inevitably never happens. These people forget about all the success stories from people just like them, while focusing only on those people that fail. All of this doubt and all of these excuses are classic symptoms of fear.

Don't wish for less problems, wish for more skills.
- JIM ROHN

Lets be real. We all know the basics of Living Lean. Eating real food and moving your body. The problem occurs when people think of all the things they must give up in order to become this healthy person. Numerous doubts cloud their thinking, fear of failure rises, and the inevitable question of "why even start?" dominates their lack of actions. Creating massive and sustainable change in your mind and body will never occur when indecision, fear, and doubt controls your mind. You must put a stop to this negative mindset now. The first step is to be aware of it. So take a few minutes right now and think about how the following questions relate to your current situation:

How do indecision, doubt, and fear affect your current outcomes?
What negative habits have they created in your life?
How are they holding you back from getting what you want?

Before you quickly pass over this exercise, I really want you to dig deep here. At first you may think none of them apply to you. Stop, take a deep breath, close your eyes, and think about each one and how you react to it. **Nice job.**

Napoleon Hill broke fear down into six different types. Even though he was referring to money, it's interesting how each one of these also applies to Living Lean.

#1. Fear of Poverty
#2. Fear of Criticism
#3. Fear of Poor Health
#4. Fear of Lost Love
#5. Fear of Old Age
#6. Fear of Death

Lets take a closer look how each one relates to Living Lean.

Fear of Poverty as it relates to Living Lean

This is a big one and I understand why. Living Lean does "cost money". I use quotes here because in a few paragraphs I'm going to explain the critical mindset shift why your health isn't a cost. But first, let me share a little story.

I've always been good with my money. I remember when I was 16 years old, I bought my first mutual fund with the money I was making from my job at the golf course. To stay on top of my investment, my mom gave me a pencil and scribbler to record the weekly price of the mutual fund I purchased. Every Tuesday I'd check it in the paper and record it in my scribbler. I thank my mom for helping me develop this habit.

Then at 18 years old I moved away to go to university. I worked three jobs at once just to cover my tuition, rent, food, and entertainment. Needless to say, I was on a tight budget. So guess which line item on my budget was always first to be cut back? Like most people and families, it was food. I would scan the weekly grocery store flyers for deals. I lived off of $1.99 frozen dinners, bread, pasta, crackers, and ramen noodles. These were essentially all the cheapest foods I could find. I looked at food as being an expense and focused on making it as small of a cost at the end of the month as possible. When I was under my food budget I celebrated. As you can tell, I had a completely different mindset back then compared to today. Sure I was doing what most college kids did. I didn't have a lot of money so I needed to stretch it as far as possible. So with that mindset you'd think this would crossover to other items on my budget. Wrong. Was I buying the cheapest beer I could find? No. Was I buying the cheapest pair of jeans and sneakers. No.

So why was I so focused on keeping my food expenses low, but was spending more freely on other things? Simple. My focus and priorities were elsewhere. My goal was to wear cool clothes so I would fit in at school. My goal was not to be as fit and healthy as possible.

Fast forward 15 years and my priorities, focus, and goals are now different. I've made being healthy a top priority in my life. So rather than buying expensive jeans just to look more stylish, I prefer to buy "more expensive" food so I can be more fit. What I'm trying to say is, look at your spending habits and you will quickly find out where your true priorities are. I always laugh when people tell me they can't afford to buy meat, vegetables, nuts, seeds, and fruit, yet they can afford $200 jeans, a premium vehicle, a big screen TV, and more channels than you can count. As a society, why are we willing to buy and eat the cheapest forms of food, yet we're not willing to buy cheaper clothing, a used vehicle, or a smaller TV? Once again, the answer is it comes down to what your priorities are.

On my Live Lean TV show, we often share videos of the foods we purchase from the grocery store and the meals we make at home. A few of the main comments we consistently receive are:

"I can't afford to eat food like that."
"Why is it so expensive to eat healthy?"

Most people focus on the extra expenses to Live Lean. The additional expense of purchasing real food vs. fake food from a box. The expense of a gym membership or buying home gym equipment. The expense of supplements. The expense of new workout clothes and sneakers. I could go on and on. And to be honest, besides the additional expense of eating real food, most of the other added expenses can be minimal. Although I highly recommend a gym membership, you can get away without having one. Even if you don't want to buy any home gym equipment, you can use your body as your barbell. You can use nature as your treadmill. I have countless videos on Live Lean TV showing you how to do this. When it comes to supplements, they're a nice to have, but not a necessity to Live Lean. I'd rather see you putting more money towards your food rather than supplements. Supplements are just that. They supplement your diet when needed, but should never be the first change made to your nutrition. And lastly, new workout clothes and sneakers can be a great motivator to get you moving, but once again, that's just a nice-to-have. You can still get in an incredible workout in old shorts and a t-shirt.

The point is, you need to make a mindset shift. Stop looking at your health and wellness as an expense. Look at it as an investment. Let me ask you this. When you're buying stocks, mutual funds, and bonds for your retirement, do you look at that as an expense? Probably not. You look at it as an investment in the wellbeing of your future. So why is your health any different? Without your health, you won't have a future! Starting today, look at your grocery receipt as your weekly investment statement of your health. All the healthy foods with minimal ingredients are appreciating assets. All the unhealthy processed foods are expenses that are eating away at your bottom line (i.e. your health). Look at your gym membership, your workout programs, your trainer, etc. as an investment that is providing compound interest in the way of years of an extended and healthy life.

Besides, think of all the money you'll be saving later in life by not having to spend it on cancer and disease treatments and medication. I don't know about you, but I plan to be spending the later years of my life living it up on the beach, not on a hospital bed.

It's all about perception. What lens are you looking through when you're deciding if something is an expense or an investment? It's a tough mindset shift, but it's a game changer.

Fear of Criticism

Fear of criticism is a major deterrent for people looking to change. It's a very uncomfortable situation when you've decided to change your poor lifestyle habits while the people around you haven't. Fear of criticism often destroys initiative, focus, drive, and taking action. It's everywhere. Often the people closest to you are the ones dishing it out the most. Even though my old friends didn't know it, every time they poked fun at me when I decided to order water rather than a beer, or a salad instead of a cheeseburger, it really made me feel uncomfortable to be around them. Maybe I was too sensitive, but the point is, criticism is poison when it's not constructive or done in a way to help you improve. It's up to you to be strong and block criticism during your journey.

Fear of Poor Health

The road to Living Lean and the road to poor health flow in opposite directions. To Live Lean, you must first refuse to accept any and all ideas of living a life of poor health. As discussed in earlier chapters, the beginning point of your journey to Live Lean is desire. If you truly desire this change in lifestyle you must declare right now that you refuse to accept anything less than a life of Living Lean. This is incredibly important. When I made that declaration, and put my money where my mouth was, everything fell into place. Failure is not an option. As I said before, burn the boat. Although you will have challenging days during your journey, deep down you will know you are progressively moving in the right direction. If you want to Live Lean, be very clear on what Living Lean means to you. Go back to your WHY as we outlined in section one. Decide exactly what that means. How many pounds of fat do you want to lose? How many pounds of muscle do you want to build? What specific size of clothing do you want to fit in? Review this vision daily. It's up to you to start this journey and continue it. If you don't complete the exercises at the end of every chapter, it's a sign that your desire is not yet strong enough to evoke the changes required to Live Lean. It's time to take a long look in the mirror. You need to take personal responsibility for where you currently are in life. If you fail, there are no excuses. You either need this or your don't. You are in control of creating the mindset necessary to Live Lean. Fear of poor health is nothing more than a state of mind. This fear can destroy all hope if you don't take action on it. You have it within you to turn that fear into action. Use that fear to drive you to make changes and become the person you deserve to be.

Fear of Love Loss

This is a tough one. Often times in a relationship, one partner is willing to change while the other is not. Now I don't claim to be a relationship expert, but I can speak from experience that you should never force your new lifestyle on a loved one that is not ready for it. This can often lead to arguments, resentment, criticism, and potentially loss of love. My only advice to you is to just be aware. Keep an open communication with your loved one about WHY it is necessary for you to make the necessary lifestyle changes. Discuss that you want to live a long life together, that you want to set a positive example for your kids, and that you want to be able to play with your grandchildren. Start slow with your loved one and be considerate. Only that person can truly commit when they have decided they need to change. The goal is to lead by example via actions and results, not by words. Over time, the hope is that your loved one will see the positive changes you've made, be inspired by you, and prepare to join you.

Fear of Death

Often times the fear of an early death motivates people to create lifestyle changes. Other times, people just accept the fact that we're all going to die sometime. And it's true, you could be the healthiest person in the world and accidentally get hit by a car tomorrow. So we need to find a balance of living a healthy lifestyle while having fun in life. Don't be one of those health perfectionists that actually causes more harm and stress to their body by trying to be perfect. In other words, eating 100% organic, never cheating on your diet, always looking for the optimal diet, etc. There's a term for this. It's called orthorexia. These people have an extreme obsession with only eating foods that are 100% optimally healthy.

When I first started Living Lean I had a little taste of this. Nothing major, but just a smidgen. I remember I had a personal goal of living to 120 years old. I read somewhere that in a perfect world, this was the age our bodies were genetically designed to live too. I wanted to be that person. However, I no longer have that goal. Why? It's simple. Living Lean is not about being perfect. It's about taking a few simple disciplined steps everyday. I accept the fact that I will have days where I don't feel like eating healthy. Therefore as long as I've been consistent with healthy eating and working out for the majority of the week, I'll have a cheat meal. I won't beat myself up about it. I don't allow myself to fall into the trap of having one cheat meal turn into a cheat week. This is because I know it's a planned meal that I earned.

I personally don't fear death. I just want to live a life where I feel good about myself, I'm confident, and I'm serving others with my message. If I die at 77. I'm okay with that. If I die at 120, then I sure hope my loved ones make it with me because it would be an awful lonely 30 years without my wife. Don't fear death. Don't try to be perfect. Just be consistent and live a life of meaning. Be grateful for every day you wake up, and be the best version of yourself. As the famous quote goes: "Life is not measured by the number of breaths we take, but by the moments that take your breath away." That's enough for me.

Failure

Failure is another killer of future progress and ambition. This unsettled state of mind is usually caused by indecision and driven by fear. The inability to make decisions and having the willpower to stick with them is often a failure point for people looking to Live Lean. Think about it. You decide on Sunday night that you're going to go to the gym Monday morning. You end up getting to the gym, slave yourself on the cardio machine for 2 hours, then head to work. By the time you get home, you're exhausted and can't imagine doing it all over again. You worry that you don't have the time or energy to continue to do it. Overtime this worry continues to build up inside of you and eventually puts a halt on any future progress and ambition.

All the fears I talked about previously are based on indecision. It's up to you to make a decision and stick with it. Make the decision that nothing in life is worth the issues that worry creates. Stop worrying about how it'll all work out. If you fill your mind with fear, you're self sabotaging all efforts to Live Lean. Your negative thoughts are creating your negative outcomes. Remember, worry can be controlled. You are in control of your mind and have the power to feed it whatever you want. Free yourself from worry of failure by focusing on trusting the process. Believe in yourself and your abilities. And take persistent action towards your goals.

LIVE LEAN ACTION STEPS

Here are your action steps to begin unlocking your strong belief in your abilities and overcoming your past failures.

ACTION STEP #1: BELIEF FORMULA

Deep inside of you, you have the potential for greatness. I truly believe that. But the problem is your greatness remains hidden and locked away inside of you. Does this mean it's lost forever? Fortunately no. Your greatness can be sparked and awakened inside of you. Easier said than done but that's what this book is about. For some unexplained reason, it's become a part of human nature for the vast majority of the population to inundate their minds with negative self-talk. As we learned earlier, the subconscious mind, the factory that turns thoughts into reality, cannot filter between positive and negative thoughts. Therefore, if your thoughts are filled with an "I'm not good enough" belief, your subconscious mind will go to work to make that a reality. In order to overcome these self-defeating thoughts, we must feed our mind with positive statements that strengthen our beliefs in our abilities. As mentioned so many times throughout this book, your thoughts create your outcomes. It's essential to build up a strong belief in your abilities. To do that, fill in the blanks and review the following statements daily:

I know I have the ability to achieve _____
_____ (write your burning goal).

I promise and demand of myself to take persistent, continuous action towards achieving _____ everyday.

I understand and take full responsibility that the dominating thoughts of my mind will either take me closer to or further away from achieving _____.

I promise to invest 30 minutes a day concentrating on positive thoughts and creating a positive vision of the person I intend to become.

I promise to invest 10 minutes a day in building my self-confidence by reviewing my list of accomplishments and continually writing new ones daily.

I am committed to building my self-confidence everyday, as I know it's critical to achieving _____

I fully realize achieving _____ will be a challenge, so I will seek out and surround myself with other like-minded, positive, and supportive people who believe in me. In return, I promise to be supportive of others, and pass on the knowledge I learn along the way to help others achieve their goals.

I commit to memorize and repeat these statements once a day, with full belief that they will influence my self-confidence, thoughts, and actions that I will achieve _____.

By signing below, I'm committing to the statements above.

_____

Signature

ACTION STEP #2: MAKE A LIST OF YOUR LIFE WINS

To start, write down as many of your wins from your life as you can think of. Then every night, continue to add to the list by writing down your wins of the day. As a recap, here are a few of my big and little wins from my journal.

- Paid my way through university and graduated debt-free
- Became a full-time entrepreneur
- Published a book
- Won the MVP award in my football league
- Set a new personal best with my deadlift
- Replied to an email from a stranger named Jessica Rumbaugh on December 31, 2012 (my fave win)
- Prepped my meals for the next 3 days.

Your list of "Life Wins" will be a lifeline to your goals when you begin to doubt your abilities. Promise me you'll implement this habit into your daily routine.

ACTION STEP #3: IMAGINE YOUR VISION STATEMENT

Since this is so important, I'm repeating the same action step from section one. To help strengthen your belief, you need to practice it. So once again, commit to memorizing and visualizing your vision statement every morning and night.

SECTION FOUR
CREATING YOUR LIFE-LONG HABITS

CHAPTER 4.1

READY, SET, ACTION

You only have control over three things in life -
the thoughts you think, the images you visualize,
and the actions you take (your behavior).
- *JACK CANFIELD*

Ready, set, ACTION! This statement is used in the movie industry all the time. A movie production can have the budget, the best written script, the best actors, but without the final piece, there are no results. And yes, that final piece is called, action. Unlike what you may have been exposed to in other best-selling books, I do not buy into the hype that you can make your desires come true by simply sitting at home thinking about them. As you've read in the previous chapters, I do see value in it, but not unless it's followed up with action. And I'm not just referring to action as following a 6 week workout program or a 30 day diet. I'm talking about taking action on creating sustainable positive habits that last a lifetime. Not a short-term fad diet or workout program to lose weight fast. This is the Live Lean lifestyle. By reading this book, you're making the incredible decision to take control of your health, 365 days a year. Action is essential to this and is something we need to ingrain into your daily behaviors.

It all starts with the first step. That's it. One step. But I also know one thing is inevitable for 80% of you. Once you do take that first step, then another, and another, some of you will then hit a wall. They'll be plenty of times you'll want to give up. In the beginning, there will be times when your results just don't seem to be happening as fast as you'd like. I get it. I've been there. But trust me, it takes time. It compounds little by little with every action step taken. You may not even realize it, but every workout and every healthy meal is intensifying your goal in your mind to Live Lean. During this time, it's critical to stay open to it and trust the process even when it gets difficult and you feel like no changes are happening to your body. The worst thing you can do is give up and lower your standards. Remember, avoid the plague of feeding a failure conscious mind by thinking thoughts of, "It's just not in the cards for me" or "I'll just have to accept my poor health situation." Wrong. That's a weak cop out. You're better than that. When you're faced with that decision, I want you to say to yourself, "I started the journey to Live Lean, and I'm going to continue to accomplish it no matter what." As I've mentioned countless times throughout this book, when times get tough, go back to your Why, your purpose, and re-focus.

A lot of times these temporary defeats are disguised as stepping-stones to opportunity. I want to ensure you rise up, and see these situations for what they really are. It's just a test. When you are truly ready for it, the Live Lean switch will turn on and your workouts and healthy eating choices will become a habit. Now when I say habit, I'm obviously referring to it as a positive habit. Habits can be either positive or negative. Unfortunately up to this moment, when it comes to your health, most of your daily habits may have been negative. On the positive side, you're now aware of this and you're ready to take action and transform.

Temporary defeats can also be caused by falling into

a rut. If you're reading this book, I'd be willing to bet most of you may be in this rut right now. Success and failure come down to habits. Poor habits lead to failure. Positive habits lead to success. In other words, over the past few days, weeks, months, or years you've accepted your less than ideal daily behaviors. This acceptance has led to your behaviors becoming formed as habits. These poor habits become so strong, and ingrained into your daily routine, you feel like you can never turn back. You show me failure, and I'll show you a person with poor habits. You show me success, and I'll show you a person with positive habits. Living Lean is all about creating and sustaining positive lifestyle habits.

Once these habits are instilled, the results will come much faster, so much so, that you'll be amazed at how quickly they come compared to when you first started your journey. Trust the process. I'll say it again, Living Lean begins with a vision, a belief, a positive mindset, a burning desire, persistence, and daily action. As soon as you master these steps, and apply them, your journey to Live Lean will be on autopilot.

Since nothing worthwhile ever comes easy, one of the most common failures people make is giving up when faced with a temporary set back. Please remember this key point. Often times people give up just when they're about to have a major breakthrough. This happened with my journey to Live Lean, and it also happened in my career. As I mentioned earlier, I was about to give up my commitment to working out and eat healthy. Luckily, before I quit, I decided to invest in expert help. Make sure you do the same before ever giving up! I remember saying to myself, I'm going to put my money where my mouth is and invest in coaching. If this fails, I'm done. I'm glad to say, the rest is history.

And even more dramatic, when it came to my entrepreneurial career in fitness, I almost gave up numerous times. As I mentioned, in my first two years of being a fitness entrepreneur, I made less than $10,000 a year in income. Of that $10,000, less than $2,000 of it came from pursuing my real purpose, my online business. The majority of my pitiful earnings came from training clients in person. Now don't get me wrong, it was great to help those clients transform their lives, but I knew my vision was to take my mission on a grander platform. My mission was to train the world.

With that said, how many of you would have given up after two years of making less than $2.30 an hour? That's right, a university graduate in business, with 8 years of corporate marketing experience, making less than $10,000 a year, or the equivalent of $2.30 an hour (or less) when you factor in how many hours I worked. Two straight years of this while losing my house, losing my wife and best friend, and feeling lost in the world! But just when I was considering giving up on my vision, I was persistent and kept going. Because of that persistence, I'm much more comfortable financially now and I truly feel like the sky is the limit.

Remember, the most successful people in the world from Steve Jobs to Thomas Edison have been faced with many temporary defeats and failures. The easiest thing to do when faced with these challenges is to give up. Unfortunately, that's what most people do. They quit when the going gets tough. That's why so many people fail to Live Lean. Failure is one sneaky S.O.B. with a love for irony. Failure loves to defeat you at time when success is just around the corner. Always believe your successful breakthrough is just one step past your current obstacles. Never stop 3 feet from striking gold. Never give up on your Why, your purpose, and your mission to Live Lean, no matter how tough it may be.

If you're one of those people that says you can't do it because you were born with bad genetics, you're absolutely right. Do I believe you can't do it? No, but it doesn't matter what I think. You're in charge and create your own world. Whether you say you can or you can't, you're always right. When you say you can, you open up your body to opportunity, when you say you can't, you've already given up. You're responsible for your life. Yes it's true, there are people born with superior genetics to you. However it's also true there are people born with worse genetics than you but are producing fantastic results by taking action.

The time is now. I'm serious. Don't wait for tomorrow. Don't wait for the weekend to get over. And please, please, please don't wait for the New Year. Decide to stop procrastinating and act NOW! And no, I don't buy the label that people place on themselves such as, "I was born a procrastinator". No you weren't. You're just scared to make a decision. You're scared that that decision may take you out of your comfort zone. You're scared it may fail. So rather than putting yourself potentially in the hurt box, you decide not to act. You just put it off for another day. This is a common theme among many people that fail to live up to their potential. That's why I'm devoting an entire chapter to it because you can and you will conquer it.

After finishing this book, you will be equipped with the tools to not only make decisions quickly, but to take action on them too. I once heard a saying that what sets successful people apart from others is their ability to make decisions quickly, and change those decisions slowly, if needed. That's the opposite of most people who are slow to act on a decision but are quick to change their mind frequently when things get tough. Think about it. Which side do you fall on? Are you quick to make decisions and slow to change your mind? Or are you slow to make decisions and quick to change your mind?

Here's an example. You know you want to Live Lean, but you don't know where to start. Do you spend week after week sitting on your butt listening to opinions on the best workout programs and meal plans? Or do you find someone you trust, and make the decision to take action right away by purchasing their program that is suitable to your goals? Be honest. Which approach have you taken in the past? Further to this, once you finally invest in the program, do you follow it for the first two days, then quickly decide it's too tough so you stop and go back to doing nothing? Or do you stay focused, persevere, and push yourself through the entire program? Remember, the workout program you don't do, won't help.

Based on these examples, which person do you think is more likely to Live Lean? It's just another classic example of how building the right mindset and taking consistent action is critical to reaching your goals. And don't get me wrong, I'm not perfect. In fact, I have many examples of making these same mistakes. I continuously fell under the "analysis paralysis" spell because I was afraid to act. For example, I knew I needed to move from my hometown to a bigger city, but I was afraid to fail. Therefore, I kept delaying taking action on the decision. I found myself listening to other people's opinions on why it wasn't a good move. This negative self-talk kept creeping into my mind. What if I can't find anywhere to live? What if I couldn't afford it? What if I can't make new friends? What if I don't like it? The "what if" questions kept piling on.

But guess what? After finally having the courage to make the decision and believing that it would work, all the "what ifs" disappeared. Other people's opinions that were holding me back didn't matter in the end. I literally arrived in my new city with one suitcase. I didn't even have an apartment or any leads. For the first two nights I stayed in a hotel. The third night, I was sleeping in my apartment. It was the first and only place I looked at, and it was perfect. Although I had some lonely nights in my new city, I stuck to my decision to stay and it all worked out in the end. Although I'm still a work in progress, with practice and consistent action, I'm much better at being quick and decisive and slower to change my decisions, if needed.

So do yourself a favor and block out the opinions of the masses. We all have a friend that always seems to knows best. They do all the talking, very little listening, yet they are living well below their potential. Don't share your vision and goals with these kinds of people. When it comes to this, I like living by the following wise words: *Don't talk about what you intend to do…show them what you DID do.* In other words, actions are stronger than words. Those who make decisions and know what they want, more often than not, get it. As a society we're too easily influenced by people who are not living the life you want. Unfortunately in many cases, these people may include family members. Have the courage to let them gossip all they want. Look at it as envy, not truth. Allow this envy to drive you. Just don't let those opinions affect your decision making. The only opinions that matter are yours, and people who you respect and look up too. This is an important reason why having a community comprised of people who have the same goals as you is so important.

When I decided to hire my first online fitness coach, I didn't tell anyone about it other than my girlfriend, who thankfully was very supportive. I can just imagine what would have happened if I told my friends that I transferred over $600 to a complete stranger online that lived over 5000 miles away, in a different country. They would have thought it was the dumbest way to spend a lot of money since there were thousands of free workouts online. Back then I was very impressionable, lacked confidence, and probably would have been swayed not to invest in myself had I told them. Who knows where I'd be now if I didn't have the courage to make that decision. I'd bet I'd still be a shy, skinny fat guy living in the same city I grew up in, working a 9-5 office job, and living well below my potential. Thankfully I had the courage to make the scary decision to invest in myself even when it may have seemed crazy to others.

Don't be scared to be the leader of your life. Have the courage to use your actions, not your words, to show other people that you know what you want and that you will do what is necessary to obtain it.

CHAPTER 4.2

GROWING WILLPOWER AND REFUSING TO QUIT

Energy and persistence conquer all things.
- *Benjamin Franklin*

If you pick up one thing from this book, it's this. To make Living Lean your reality, it requires a strong willpower and ongoing persistent action. There's no way around it, persistence is king. Without persistence, you've failed before you even started. Lets be real, Living Lean is not easy. If it was, everyone would be doing it. And it's definitely not about taking shortcuts to reach your destination as fast as possible. Don't get me wrong, fast is great as long as it's safe and sustainable. But unfortunately when it comes to health and fitness, fast shortcuts usually mean unsafe and short-term.

Think about the last great thing that happened in your life. Maybe it was getting a raise, or meeting the girl of your dreams. Did you acquire this easily? Or did it take willpower, ongoing persistence, and effort? Living Lean is no different. It's not about how fast you can get there. It's about how you can consistently show up day after day, even when you don't feel like it. It's about having the willpower to walk away from the things in life that are taking you away from your goals. Next time you think you're hungry at night, and I say "think" because you're really just bored, do you grab a bag of potato chips or do you have a cup of tea? You know the right answer. But the question is, do you have the willpower and focus to be persistent in your journey towards your goals? Or are you going to continuously allow temporary setbacks to get in your way? You have the choice. No one is shoving this food into your mouth. You either want it, or you don't. Be the type of person that acknowledges these minor setbacks or defeats as what they are. Temporary. Commit right now, to never allow yourself to look at defeats as permanent. When you have a burning desire, any defeat, with persistence, can be turned into a victory. Too many people want to be healthy, but when they're faced with a bad day of eating, they let that temporary defeat keep them down for good. The people who are Living Lean, still face the same setbacks that you do, the difference is they're persistent in getting back up every time. That's the key ingredient in the secret sauce of uber successful people. Read any autobiography on game changing individuals, and you'll see a common trait. They fail many times, but no matter how many times they do, they keep getting back up. Think about the countless actors who were rejected and told no a thousand times before hearing one yes that changed their lives. They refused to quit. Persistence was the trait behind all of these success stories.

I've trained numerous clients with different backgrounds in my day. Business executives, doctors, engineers, administrative 9-5'ers, students, etc. Guess which client I enjoyed training the most? The business executives. Why? It was simple. They were persistent. When the reps began to burn, they kept fighting through. When they wanted to stop sprinting, they realized the finish line was only 20 meters away so they dug deeper and ran even faster. It's no surprise to me that these people were also successful in business. Like the old saying goes, "When the going gets tough, the tough gets going". The principles of persistency crosses all borders when it comes to success in life. Those who have it or developed it, are rewarded with the goal they desire.

To date I've received so many incredible Live Lean before and after transformations from people just like you. Besides the trait of persistent action, they also hung out and received support from like-minded people. Never forget, the beginning point of success and creating willpower always starts with a vision, desire, and a emotional Why. Strong desires create strong results. Weak desires create weak results.

So if you're lacking persistence and constantly finding yourself faltering and quitting your journey to Live Lean, I'll say it again, go back to your Why. Why is your goal important? What will happen to you if you continue to quit and never achieve it? Many people who have taken control back of their health did it out of necessity. Their doctor's told them, if you don't do "x", "y" will happen. This scare tactic quickly enabled them to create the habit of persistency. This is why emotional connections to your goals and desires are so important. They are the driving power behind strengthening your "persistency muscles".

AMBITION is the path to success,
PERSISTENCE is the vehicle you arrive in.
- WILLIAM EARDLEY

CHAPTER 4.3

STAYING IN THE ZONE FOR LIFE

Persistence and determination alone are omnipotent.
The slogan 'press on' has solved and always will
solve the problems of the human race.
- *CALVIN COOLIDGE*

Negative influences are like a cancer to your journey to Live Lean. When I'm referring to negative influences, I'm not only talking about outside influences. I'm also speaking to the self-served influences you feed your mind every day. As mentioned throughout this book, developing the Live Lean Mindset is about self-discipline and creating daily positive habits. These habits are formed to stay in the zone and focus on taking persistent action towards your goals. This leaves no room for negative influences. Ask yourself right now, how well do you react to negative influences. Are you resilient and stick to your goals? Or do you allow yourself to be defeated in the face of temptation?

If I haven't said it enough already, let me say it again.

You are in control of one of the most important things on your journey to Live Lean, your thoughts. You have the willpower to protect yourself and overcome any internal or external negative influence. It will be difficult in the beginning, but over time, when you get into the habit of flexing your willpower, it will continue to grow stronger. Flexing your willpower and owning your thoughts will allow you to stay in the zone and accomplish major things not only with your body, but also your life. Your mind and body are the most valuable pieces of real estate you will ever own. Put in the work. Protect it, nurture it, and flourish.

One way to ensure you stay in the zone is by focusing on hanging out with people who uplift you and support you towards your goals. Close your mind from negative influences. Distance yourself from the energy zapping zombie's who do nothing but criticize and bring you down. Many people don't realize how the people around them are influencing their current situation. Although you need to take personal responsibility for yourself, you can do this by making tough decisions. This may seem difficult, but it's a game changer. To change your future, you must change your today. This may mean leaving behind negative influences and people in your life. Hard stuff, but sometimes it's necessary.

When I made the transition from the corporate world to an entrepreneurial lifestyle, many people in my circle thought I was crazy. I experienced a lot of negativity from people with their limiting thoughts on what was possible. Some people close to me just didn't believe I could survive on my own. The conversations were always uncomfortable and I knew the criticism was beating me down. So I made the decision to change my surroundings. I decided to associate myself with people who are also creating the lifestyle that I was searching for. This tough action had an amazing transformation on my mindset. By associating myself with other success stories, I realized that it was possible. If they could do it, why not me? I saw an opportunity, and created it by consistently working my butt off. Like Napoleon Hill said, anything the mind could conceive and believe, it could achieve. Associating with other like-minded people helped me believe that I could do it too. The same applies for your journey to Live Lean. Clear your mind of negative influences.

Also, if you expect bad things to happen, they will. Always think that things will work out for you. When I look back at all the changes that have happened to me over the past 4 years, one thing remains constant. No matter how bad it may have seemed at the time. Things have always worked out for me in the end. My heart breaking divorce created the opportunity for me to meet my beautiful wife Jessica. It also allowed me to follow my dream and move to Los Angeles. After firing my boss in 2011, I was making less than $3 and hour as an entrepreneur. My business is now flourishing with new opportunities arising every day. Think positively about your workouts. Think optimistically about your nutrition. And always think, no matter how much you're struggling with your current lifestyle changes, if you persistently work at it, it'll always work out over time.

When things get tough, the excuses follow. Do not fall for the excuse mindset. Now is not the time for excuses. I hear from countless people everyday talking about why they can't Live Lean. Even if they haven't yet taken the first step, they list all the reasons why they're bound to fail. In other words, they're creating their destiny before even trying. Excuses are the poison that will keep you from staying in the zone. In the action steps to follow, I'm going to list 25 of the most common excuses when it comes to Living Lean. Make note of how many of these you have used, then commit to erasing them from your mindset. Using excuses to explain why you're not getting the results you want is disastrous to your journey to Live Lean. Stop the excuses right now. They aren't real. You are the one who is making them up to cover weaknesses in your life. It's time to confront your weaknesses and turn them into strengths. Focus on spending your time on improving your weaknesses rather than building them up via more excuses.

CHAPTER 4.4

FOLLOWING THE LIVE LEAN FORMULA

Don't let your learning lead to knowledge.
Let your learning lead to action.
- JIM ROHN

How many of you have heard the saying, "Knowledge is power"? Raise your hand and say, "Yeeeeeep" (don't worry know one is looking). Alright now let me ask, how many of you believe this saying is true? I'm sure most of you would agree. Me? Not so much. Here's why. Most people know that in order to lose weight they have to exercise and eat healthy. In other words, 95.67% of adults have the knowledge that to lose weight you need to burn more calories than you eat. So if 95.67% of adults have this knowledge, why is up to 70% of the population in the United States overweight? The answer is simple. I believe knowledge gives us the potential for power, but it's just one part of the overall equation. Knowledge becomes power once it's organized into a plan of action directed towards obtaining an end goal. No plan of action. No power.

You can be the smartest person in the world. You may understand the biology, the anatomy, and the physiology, but if you don't have a plan and more importantly, take action on it, all the knowledge in the world won't help you Live Lean. I don't know about you, but I've seen many highly educated, but overweight doctors, personal trainers, and nutritionists. These people obviously have the knowledge, but they lack a plan and action. Knowledge is absolutely useless to Living Lean unless it's organized into a plan of action directed towards obtaining an end goal.

This is why I'm always stressing the importance of investing in a workout program. All of our Live Lean programs take the knowledge required to lose weight or build muscle and organize it into an actionable plan. All the knowledge of building effective workout program design protocols has already been done for you. The action plan has been put in place for you. Now all you need to do is take action on the plan and workout. Doesn't that sound a lot better than being that guy who walks into the gym, empty handed, blindly staring at the machines, scratching his head, and trying to figure out what he should do today? I see multiple types of those guys and girls every workout. And if I just described you, don't feel bad. 10 years ago I used to be that guy. I may have had enough general knowledge to think I could do it on my own, but what I lacked was the specialized knowledge of how to design an effective workout program using protocols that were suited to my goals. In other words, I possessed general knowledge (enough to be dangerous), I was taking action, but I was missing the third piece of the power equation, a specialized plan.

The key takeaway from this story is to know your limits. It's not required that you possess the specialized fitness and nutrition knowledge to Live Lean. What is required to turn your burning desire into reality, is having access to, and taking action on a specialized plan that is designed to help you reach your specific goal of Living Lean. Don't be stubborn like I was. Don't try to do it yourself. The same principles apply in business, especially with new entrepreneurs like myself. Rather than trying to become an expert in every aspect of my business, i.e. website design, IT programming, graphic design, etc., I've learned it's much more effective to build a team of experts and hire out the specialized skills.

When it comes to your health, and Living Lean, I highly recommend you do the same. Save yourself a lot of time and frustration and invest in a professional program. Not only will results come a lot faster, but when you have "skin in the game" (in the form of money invested in the program), you're more likely to complete the program through to the end. New habits will be formed and new goals will be reached. Doesn't that sound a lot better than being that dude who invests hundreds of dollars in a gym membership, then disappears after the first few weeks due to lack of results or not having a clue of what to do?

Have you hit your turning point yet? That moment in time when you clearly decided that you were committed to making a change. It could be related to your health, your career, or your personal relationships. I've experienced them all. As I just mentioned, the most critical turning point with my health came in February of 2010. I was super frustrated. I was "working hard", but obviously based on my lack of results, I wasn't working smart. 1-2 years before reaching my turning point, I remember cutting and pasting all the workouts and recipes every month from my favorite fitness magazine into a binder. Then I'd randomly follow whatever workout I felt like doing. That of course, turned into many less effective "mirror muscle" workouts. I'd also end up eating a lot of recipes featuring "advertiser of the month" foods that were filled with processed ingredients. Even after 1-2 years of consistent "workouts and healthy eating", I still wasn't where I wanted to be. Then I read the famous definition of insanity quote from Einstein: *"Doing the same thing over and over again yet expecting different results."* That was my turning point. I realized if

I wanted to change, I needed to change my approach to fitness and nutrition. As I've mentioned before, that led me to seek out and invest in a program from a coach that was getting the results I wanted.

Bottom line. At the time, my "general knowledge" of fitness and nutrition actually hindered my progress. I thought I knew enough to do it on my own. Luckily I took the risk and invested in specialized help. Now I realize the most successful people in the world have reached those levels by surrounding themselves with people and resources that have specialized knowledge in specific areas. These successful people don't try to be a master of all domains. If your goal is to build a beautiful and safe home, you would probably invest in hiring a proven architect to design the plans for your home. Likewise, if your goal is to build a strong, lean, and healthy body, doesn't it also make sense to invest in the specialized knowledge from a proven fitness trainer? Your health should be your priority. So why are you investing in materialistic things but not your own body? Consider your fitness trainer as just another specialist in your life's "mastermind" group, along with your banker, your tax advisor, your electrician, your hair stylist, etc. With this chapter, I hope I've opened your eyes to the fact that you may need assistance from someone with specialized knowledge to help you Live Lean.

My education in fitness and health did not stop with that first investment in coaching. I also went on to study towards my professional certifications in fitness training as well as nutrition and wellness coaching. Once I received those certifications, I continued reading books and attending seminars from the top fitness and nutrition coaches in the world. Increasing your knowledge doesn't stop after you get your degree, certification, or license. The most successful professionals never stop learning. So if you're an up and coming health professional that just received your certifications, your learning has just begun. However, if health and fitness is not your career and it's not your passion, once again, I highly recommend you focus your time and effort on what you love and are specialized in. Rather than writing your own workout and nutrition plans, I highly recommend you invest in a fitness professional and add them to your life's mastermind group. As mentioned earlier, don't look at your health as an expense. Look at your gym membership, your trainer, and healthy food as an investment towards a life of health. It's all about your priorities. I'm always floored when people say they can't afford a trainer, yet I see them driving an expensive car. They say they can't afford healthy food, yet I see them wearing $200 sneakers. Most people can find the money to invest in their health, but unfortunately they're priorities and actions aren't inline with their desired outcomes. If your burning desire really is to Live Lean, don't make the same mistake. Make the commitment to invest in your health.

LIVE LEAN ACTION STEPS

Just like Living Lean is made up of various daily habits, persistence can also be developed into a habit. This is made possible by:

1. Having a clear goal and a strong emotional connection to why that goal is important.
2. Having an organized and proven plan of action to accomplish that goal.
3. Having a supportive group of like-minded individuals to fuel your mind with reasons why it can be done. It's important to do your best to block all negative and discouraging influences from your daily interactions.

Can you see how those three topics, when put to work, can help you accomplish anything you desire in life? Persistence is what keeps you moving forward. It's what keeps you getting up time and time again after life knocks you down. It's what all great leaders and successful people have in common. It's not education. It's not money. It's not luck. These high achievers have persistence towards accomplishing a specific goal.

Life doesn't give you what you need,
life gives you what you deserve.
- JIM ROHN

Without applying the concepts discussed in this chapter, you won't move anywhere. Harsh, I know. But it's so true. You can know what to do and how to do it, but that information is absolutely useless if you don't take action and do anything about it. You'll never change. Continuous action is essential on your journey to Live Lean. There's no substitute for effort. No shortcuts around it. This chapter will help you create that action-oriented mindset.

Action is not only required to start your journey to Live Lean, it is essential for creating an on-going, long-term sustainable healthy lifestyle.

ACTION STEP #1: CREATE AN ACTION-ORIENTED MINDSET

1. **HAVING A CLEAR VISION.** As discussed earlier, when you have a clear vision of the goal you are working towards, action will follow.

2. **REFLECT ON YOUR EXPERIENCES TO DATE.** Be aware of how you feel when you look in the mirror. How does it feel when you take your shirt off at the beach or in the locker room? Now I'm not saying this to beat you up. I'm saying this to make a point. These real life pain points are prime examples that clearly show you need to make a change in your life. I've been there too. Eventually I struggled with my own self-confidence so much that I reached a boiling point. I knew I could no longer be afraid or embarrassed of my body. This self-awareness eventually drove me to take massive action and it worked.

3. **BECOME AWARE OF OTHERS.** Sometimes it takes seeing someone else struggle before you become aware of your own issues. How do you feel when you watch people wander around looking lost and confused at the gym? Do you feel the same emotional pain as them? Sometimes seeing the pain in life through someone else's eyes is what will spark a fire for you to make a change yourself.

Your action-oriented mindset may be influenced through one or all of these factors. Regardless of how many, the most important part is to become aware that change needs to occur in your life.

ACTION STEP #2: BUILDING PERSISTENT WILLPOWER

Here are 8 different points about being persistent and building willpower, including why you may be failing at each one. Make sure you study these action steps and reflect. Make notes in your journal about which ones you need to work on.

1. **YOUR WHY.** In Section One, we discussed your Why. Have you figured out your why yet? Having a strong emotional connection to your Why is the most important ingredient in developing willpower and persistence. A strong why will drive your daily behaviors to overcome any obstacle that's in your way. This then will create positive life-long habits. *Why you may be failing:* You wish you could Live Lean instead of working to make it happen. This is because you don't have a strong emotional reason to change (your Why). Therefore you're still indifferent to taking persistent action on making the necessary habitual changes needed to change your life. Until you figure out your Why, you won't be willing to compromise your current and less disciplined lifestyle.

2. **YOUR GOAL.** Do you have a clear and focused goal? Persistence comes naturally when you are sharply focused on a desired goal that is the driving force behind your Why. *Why you may be failing:* you haven't clearly defined what you want to accomplish. You lack the motivation to push yourself outside of your comfort zone in case you fail.

3. **YOUR BELIEF IN YOUR ABILITIES.** Do you believe in yourself? When you have a strong belief in your talents and abilities, persistence flows. *Why you may be failing:* You keep making excuses why you can't do it. You place the blame on everything else for why you're in this current situation rather than taking personal responsibility for the life decisions you've made to date.

4. **YOUR ORGANIZED PLAN.** Are you following a plan or program? Having a plan or program to follow is a great way to entice persistence. No guesswork required. Just action. *Why you may be failing:* You are overwhelmed with analysis paralysis thus never make a decision to start today.

In other words, you're waiting for the perfect time to start. This leads to ongoing procrastination as you don't have a plan or program to keep you accountable (or pushing you to get started).

5. **YOUR KNOWLEDGE.** Do you have the required knowledge to take action? If not, are you following a proven plan that is aligned with your goals? Similar to the organized plan, when this plan is also proven to work, it's a great way to build persistence as you know the only thing stopping you is effort. *Why you may be failing:* You don't have the required knowledge to do it yourself and you don't see the value in investing in help.

6. **YOUR SURROUNDINGS.** Do you have a support group? When you surround yourself with a supportive group of like-minded individuals, it'll help keep you focused and moving toward your goal with persistence. *Why you may be failing:* Unfortunately many people's fear of criticism is stronger than their desire for success. This is a big one because it usually involves family members and friends. You're scared of being criticized or made fun of by them. Comments such as "who do you think you are?", or "you'll never be able to stick with it" ruin your desire and confidence. These people continuously fill your head with all the reasons why it can't work. This negativity causes you to easily succumb to their peer pressure rather than stand your ground and follow through on what's best for you. You'd rather live down to the standards of the people you associate with rather than putting yourself out there and growing your circle of influence. You choose comfort and safety over risk and reward/growth.

7. **YOUR WILLPOWER.** Do you practice it? Having the willpower to consistently stay focused on your goals leads to persistence. Ask yourself this when pressed with a tough decision, "Is this going to take me closer to, or further away from my goals?". Act accordingly.

Why you may be failing: You quit every time you're faced with adversity. You prefer to stay down after a defeat rather than get up and keep moving forward.

8. **YOUR HABITS**. Are you aware of your daily habits? When you think about brushing your teeth everyday, you probably don't associate that with being persistent. But that's exactly what it is. You persistently brush your teeth before you go to bed every day. Living Lean is no different. Creating life-long habits leads to persistency. So before you say you lack persistency in life, think about the simple daily habits that you do everyday. Working out and eating healthy are no different. They are habits just like brushing your teeth. *Why you may be failing:* You continuously look for shortcuts, the quick fix, or the magic pill, rather than facing the fact that to get what you want out of life, you have to replace bad habits with good habits. There's no such thing as something for nothing.

Now that you've read these 8 points. Go back and review them to decide which ones you need to work on. Be honest with yourself. You do want to improve right? A little analysis can go a long way on your journey to Live Lean. There's no turning back now!

ACTION STEP #3: ACKNOWLEDGE & AVOID THESE EXCUSES

Do any of these common excuses sound familiar? Be honest with yourself.

1. If only my husband or wife would do it with me…
2. If only I had the money to be able to afford the food…
3. If only I had you as my personal trainer…
4. If only I had access to a better gym…
5. If only I had the energy…
6. If only I had the time to cook…
7. If only I had the time to grocery shop…

8. If only I had the time to workout…
9. If only my friends would stop making me party with them all the time…
10. If only I was younger…
11. If only I could start over again…
12. If only I wasn't afraid of what people would think of me…
13. If only I wasn't embarrassed of being in the gym…
14. If only I knew what exercises I should be doing…
15. If only I didn't have injuries…
16. If only I had friends who could help me…
17. If only I lived in a better city…
18. If only my city had access to outdoor parks and trails…
19. If only I were not so fat…
20. If only I did not have such a sugar craving…
21. If only our office had access to healthier snack options…
22. If only I had a gym closer to home…
23. If only the weather were nicer…
24. If only I wasn't so lazy…

   …and the most important one of all…

25. If only I had the courage, the self-esteem, and the ability to see my own potential, and to take personal responsibility for being where I am today, and to stop making excuses and start making changes to my daily habits. Then I would take action every day towards turning my goals and beliefs into reality.

ACTION STEP #4: BECOME AWARE OF YOUR PRIORITIES

Think about all the areas of your life where you currently invest in other people's services for their specialized knowledge. For example, it could be your bigger investments such as your real estate agent, your financial advisor, or your lawyer. It could also be smaller investments such as your hair stylist, your mechanic, or your plumber. Now I want you to think about what is most important in your life, your health.

How much are you investing in other people's specialized knowledge to help you live your healthiest life? If the answer is zero dollars, you need to re-assess your priorities and what is most important in your life.

SECTION FIVE
BUILDING YOUR ACCOUNTABILITY TEAM

CHAPTER 5.1

TAKING AN INVENTORY OF YOUR SURROUNDINGS

I found there was only one way to look thin:
hang out with fat people.
- RODNEY DANGERFIELD

For most people, this is going to be a tough chapter. Why? Well, it's time to take an objective look at the people you hang out with most. I'm sure you've heard this a million times, but studies show you either life up to or life down to the standards of the 5 people you hang out with most. I remember the first time I heard this. It was in 2007 and I was just beginning to realize I wasn't fulfilling my life's passion. In fact, at that point I wasn't even sure of what my passion was. I just knew it had something to do with being an entrepreneur rather than a corporate desk jockey. To help find my path, I invested in tickets to a business conference hosted by Donald Trump in Toronto. Even though this conference was over 7 years ago, I can still feel the contagious energy of the room. Then one of the speakers dropped the bomb on me. I can't remember what the speaker's name was, but he said, "If you are the [most ambitious] person in your group of friends, it's time to find some new friends". Wow. That one statement changed me. Note: I put brackets around the word "most ambitious" because you can insert whatever goal speaks to you. For example, you could insert healthiest, smartest, most successful, etc. You get the point.

Now don't get me wrong, if you are the most "x" of your 5 closest friends, it doesn't make your friends bad people. It just means they may not be the best influence on you to achieve your desired goal. I had a very tight group of friends that went all the way back to my days of playing hockey at the age of 5. We went to school together, we moved in together, we partied together, we pretty much did everything together. They truly were, and still are, a great group of people that would do anything for each other. However, eventually I unintentionally distanced myself from them. Now that I think about it, I just felt like I was on a different path than they were. Not better, not worse, just different. As we all entered the adult stage of our lives, we all eventually got 9-5 jobs, got married, bought homes (in the same city where we all grew up), and added dogs and kids to our families. For some reason, this settling into the comfort zone was very uncomfortable for me. As I mentioned earlier, I just felt like I was destined to follow a different path. A path that didn't include a 9-5 office job, or living in the same city for my whole life, or adding that comfort layer of grown up fat. Bottom line, even though my close friends are awesome people, I subconsciously made the decision that if I was to follow my passion, get super healthy, and create the life I was imagining, I had to let go. To be honest, I have many nights where I miss those guys like crazy. But if I stayed in that comfort zone, I'd never be fulfilling my life's purpose and dreams like I am today.

So now that you know about my experience, it's time to reflect on your current situation. Think about the 5 people you hang out with most. Are they helping you get closer to your goals or are they taking you further away from them? Are they positive people that support, encourage, and uplift you, or do they drag you down? Let me make this clear. I am not telling you to abandon your friends. All I'm suggesting is that you become aware of your surroundings, and then proceed from there.

CHAPTER 5.2

GROWING YOUR LIVE LEAN DREAM TEAM

People inspire you, or they drain you. Pick them wisely.
- *HANS F. HANSEN*

Now it's time to get further outside your comfort zone and begin to make connections with other like-minded people. When I say "like-minded" people, I'm referring to aligning yourself with a group of people that have the same goals and desires that you do. Essentially people that are committed to a journey of Living Lean.

Before you start searching for your dream team, think about how you can add value to benefit the other members of your group. Think of this group as your mastermind dream team. If you're not aware of what a mastermind is, it's a group of individuals sharing information, and working together to achieve the same purpose. Being involved in a mastermind is one sure fire way to fast track your success. Why? It's simple. It's human nature to be connected to one another. Call it what you want, but as human beings we are all spiritually connected.

When you surround yourself with like-minded people that are unified in harmony as team; it's always stronger than trying to succeed alone. Most successful people in life will quickly tell you that a team is always stronger than the individual when obtaining any goal. Like the old saying goes, two heads are better than one. Think about it. Can you imagine what kind of results and empowerment you could get if you surrounded yourself in a room filled with other determined brains? Imagine the power you'd have to achieve your goals when you associate yourself with people going through the same lifestyle changes that you are, as well as experts who know what they're doing. The increased energy, drive, passion, education, accountability, and support are unmatched. Extraordinary things can occur when you align yourself with others. You become who you hang out with most. Join a mastermind, create your own, or simply join our team of like-minded, positive Live Leaners just like you at our inner circle: TeamLiveLean.com.

Side Note: *Now I'll be honest. This idea of masterminding is still an area in my professional life that I'm working on. Although I've invested thousands of dollars in attending events, and have met many of my mentors, I'm still working towards becoming better at this principle. With that said, over the past few weeks I've been approached and agreed to join a pretty high level mastermind group of fitness professionals. The investment is high, but the return will be even greater. Don't look at the cost of a good opportunity, look at what it will cost you if you don't invest in yourself.*

If you're more of a leader, you can also look at creating your own dream team mastermind. However in order to recruit people to your dream time, you need to give people a reason to buy in to the idea. Think of it as a pitch. What value can you (and the other people in your dream team) provide to John Smith in exchange for his time and commitment? This goes the other way as well. Before inviting someone into your dream team, be sure they are also committed to providing value to other members.

Remember, quality over quantity. Living in the digital

age, we are now connected to more people than ever before. But don't fall into the trap that more is better. Focus on adding quality people that are truly dedicated to Living Lean and can provide ongoing help and support to others. Also before accepting people into your group make sure they are not quitters. You only want to spend your valuable time with winners.

"A winner never quits and a quitter never wins."

Once you have a group (or a just one buddy) in place, agree to schedule meetings at least twice a week in the beginning. You can do this online via a web conference call (i.e. Skype), or if your group is local, meet at someone's house. Keep the meetings structured with an agenda that is focused on the goal of Living Lean.

Ensure all members of the group are in alignment with the goals of the mastermind, feel safe to express their wins and failures, and are supportive and judgement-free. The cooperation and harmony of the mastermind is essential. Do not allow negativity or viruses into your mastermind. If somebody in the group seems to be thinking negatively and NOT contributing to the success of the group, take corrective action by speaking to the group, and immediately remove that person if the other members of the group are in agreement.

If you're finding the mastermind meetings aren't creating value for everyone, start over. Replace the agendas, remove non-cooperative group members, etc. Persistence is key. As Napoleon Hill once said, "…temporary defeat is not permanent failure". It simply means the current plan of action had flaws. Turn this temporary defeat into success by continually working to perfect your own mastermind plan, or search to join a dream team that already has a winning formula. Mastermind groups have been proven time and time again to be a game changer, but they must be managed properly. If you don't know how to do this or don't want to lead it, once again

I highly encourage you to join our group of like-minded Live Leaners at TeamLiveLean.com. We'd love to have you.

LIVE LEAN ACTION STEPS

ACTION STEP #1: TAKE AN INVENTORY

Start by taking 2 minutes right now and write down in your journal the 5 people you spend the most time with. These 5 people will probably include friends, co-workers, and close family members. However for this exercise, don't include anyone from your family.

1.

2.

3.

4.

5.

Now think about those 5 people and answer this question: Are they helping you get closer to fulfilling your burning desire or are they taking you further away from it? Are they supportive of your new views on living a healthy lifestyle or are they poking fun at you and using peer pressure to keep you living a "normal" life? Reflect on this. Only you will know what your next step should be.

ACTION STEP #2: CREATE OR JOIN AN EXISTING GROUP

If you don't have the time or skills to start your own support group/mastermind, join us at **TeamLiveLean.com.** You'll be joined by hundreds of other people going through the same Live Lean steps as you. You'll also be provided with new workouts, new video cooking lessons, meal plans, grocery lists, and so much more. All the work has been done for you. You just need to take action on it. Go to **TeamLiveLean.com** now.

SECTION SIX
SERVING AN ATTITUDE OF GRATITUDE

CHAPTER 6.1

ADDING IN A SERVING OF GRATITUDE

Stay strong. Stay positive. Stay grateful.
- *UNKNOWN*

There is one day out of the year that most of us focus on giving thanks and sharing how we're grateful. Thanksgiving. But more and more studies are showing how having an attitude of gratitude, 365 days a year, is linked to better health, more satisfaction in life, and more loving relationships. When all these things are in place, a life of Living Lean is just around the corner. This is why I've devoted an entire section on the power of gratitude. Gratitude is defined as "the quality of being thankful; readiness to show appreciation for and to return kindness."

Research points to the fact that our brains are not wired to make us happy. That's probably not a big surprise to you as we all have bad days where things just go wrong. We feel down on ourselves, we don't like the way we look, and our progress is moving at a snails pace. But like most things in life, we are in control by the choices we decide to make. The practice of gratitude is an excellent way to re-wire your brain to focus on what is great in your life. Gratitude is another area in my life that I'm continuously working to improve. In this chapter I want to share a few of the strategies that I use to stay grateful for everything I have in my life. Not only will this make you happier, it'll help you take action to attract more of what you want in your life.

As mentioned in section three, you should already be keeping an ongoing "Life Wins" list. Similar to this list, I want you to keep an ongoing "Gratitude List". This is a way to keep an inventory of all the things you are grateful for in your life. Every night and every morning, ask yourself, "What am I grateful for at this exact moment in time." Whatever comes to mind, add it to your list. Get super specific. Rather than just saying I'm grateful for my wife, say I'm grateful for the way my wife supports me on my journey to Live Lean. Rather than saying I'm grateful for the summer. Say I'm grateful for the early morning warm sunrises as it makes my morning walk all the more enjoyable. Here's an example of my gratitude list:

Brad's Gratitude List

1. I am grateful to live 5 minutes from the beautiful beaches in Los Angeles.
2. I am grateful to have a loving and supportive wife that I LOVE!
3. I am grateful for each and every comment on my Live Lean TV episodes.
4. I am grateful to have the energy to wake up at 5am and work on my life's mission.
5. I am grateful to workout at the world famous Gold's Gym in Venice, California.

Continuously adding new items to your Gratitude List and reviewing it daily is an ongoing habit that will change your outlook on life. This isn't just a short-term exercise for the next 30 days. Think about the impact it will have when you're always focusing on what you have versus what you lack. It will trick your brain into seeing all the successes you have in life rather than seeing all the negatives. It's also another fantastic tool to create the success conscious mindset that we talked about earlier.

Studies show that people who add to their gratitude list just once a week reported feeling happier and more optimistic than those who did not. So just imagine how you'd feel doing it every night before you close your eyes and reviewing it in the morning. It's a game changer.

If you want to sleep more soundly, count blessings, not sheep.
- DR. ROBERT EMMONS

When you're down, when it seems like your body is not progressing as fast as you want, think about all you have to be grateful about. If you have two legs, you have the ability to move your body whenever you like. Be grateful that you can breath on your own. Be grateful that you have hands to pick up a dumbbell. Just being able to afford this book, or having the skills to know how to read it, or even the vision to be able to see it, is a blessing. This all may seem basic, but the power in it is phenomenal. Gratitude is more than just a feeling. Anyone can experience it and benefit from it. It washes all the negativity away, so never forget how well you have it.

CHAPTER 6.2

BEING GRATEFUL DOESN'T MEAN SETTLING

*Wanting more doesn't mean that you're ungrateful or greedy.
It means that you acknowledge that you are the master of
your destiny.*
- JACK CANFIELD

When I was outlining the steps for this book, I knew I needed to include a section on gratitude. However, I did have one concern with including this topic. I'm talking about settling. More specifically, using the excuse of being grateful to stop you from pushing yourself outside of your comfort zone. As our Live Lean mission continues to grow, I'm hearing this more and more. People would prefer to settle with being slightly overweight rather than taking the necessary steps to becoming healthier. As mentioned throughout the book, our goal is daily progress not perfection. So I have an issue with people doing the bare minimum.

Lets take John for example. John was 250 pounds and recently lost 25 pounds of fat. For good reason, John was very excited and grateful for that progress. However, that initial 25 pounds should just be the beginning for John. Based on John's current body composition, at 6'1" and 225 pounds he is still 25 pounds overweight. However since losing the initial weight, John has become more complacent. He's noticing the fat is not burning off as fast or easy anymore. This is normal during your Live Lean journey. Fat loss is not a linear process. As you begin to burn more fat, it becomes more challenging to keep the process going forward. This is an example of John hitting a weight loss plateau. In order to break this plateau, John needs to "dial it in" more with his workouts and diet. However John is still living on his past accomplishments. He's not yet ready to take his training and diet to the next level. And when I say the next level, I'm not talking about Olympic athlete precision. I'm simply talking about taking the necessary baby steps to further coax off the body fat. Unfortunately for John, he's fine with staying in his comfort zone and not pushing his potential any further.

Does that sound familiar to you? Have you made progress, celebrated it, then fell into the complacency trap? Are you just grateful for losing some weight? If so, you're not using the power of gratitude to attract more into your life. You're using it as an excuse to be complacent. Even though you think you're being grateful, you're actually holding yourself back. You've settled. You've placed self-limitations on your potential because you're scared to fail.

Don't get me wrong. I want you to celebrate the wins during your journey. I want you to feel great about your progress. I just don't want you to stop short when you have the ability to achieve what you truly desire. Use gratitude to achieve and attract abundance in your life. Don't use it as an excuse to settle.

CHAPTER 6.3

PAYING IT FORWARD

You can have everything in life you want if
you will just help enough other people get what they want.
- ZIG ZIGLAR

What a great topic to end our Think and Live Lean journey together. Being grateful is not only about reflecting on what's great in your life. It's also about paying it forward and being generous to others. I've been hosting Live Lean TV for over 3 years now. During that time, I've built up a nice following of loyal "Live Leaners". They are not only watching the show and investing in my programs, they are also taking action and applying what they're learning. Although this is awesome, there is one more step to become a true Live Leaner. The final step is paying it forward. If you're unfamiliar with that term, it simply means teaching others what you have learned.

As I travel, I'm fortunate to meet many of you at the airport, in gyms, and at our Live Lean meet ups. One of my favorite things is hearing about your Live Lean success stories. I recently met a really nice guy at one of our New York City meet ups in Central Park. He was an awesome dude and very grateful for all the things he's learned from me. Although I have to bring up one thing he said that bothered me. Like I always do, I always ask people to share our message with others. When we have as big of a mission as we do, to transform the lives of 1,000,000 people, it takes a nation, the Live Lean Nation, to make it happen. However, after this guy was done sharing how grateful he was for everything I do, I thanked him, and asked him if he's been sharing our videos with others. His response shocked me. He said he doesn't share our videos because he wants to keep me as his secret Live Lean weapon. In other words, he didn't want other people, or his competition (as he saw it), having the same access to this information as he had. He looked at it as being his competitive advantage.

As we light a path for others, we naturally light our own way.
- MARY ANNE RADMACHER

Now don't get me wrong, for someone to think of my teachings as a secret weapon, it makes me feel pretty special. But just like it's your duty as a Live Leaner to take action on working out and eating healthy, it's also your final duty to pay it forward by teaching someone else. In fact, there are several studies that show the best way to learn something is to teach it to others. Paying it forward, spreading the message, and ultimately helping other people is one of the most powerful ways to ensure you truly are committed to this new Live Lean Mindset. In a sense, it's one of the main reasons why I wanted to write this book. As I've mentioned many times already, I've applied every principle in this book to my own life. I've been grateful to reap the success from it, but my ultimate sense of empowerment comes from teaching what I've learned to others. I want you to experience that same sense of empowerment that I feel. You are now knowledgeable, you have the abilities, and helping others will give you a greater sense of purpose and self-worth. I promise, if you accept this challenge to pay it forward, you will be taking one of the most positive actions you can in continually growing a stronger Live Lean Mindset.

Do you see how this mindset shift not only dramatically improves your life, but also the life of someone else? It's more fun when all your friends and family are fit than when you're the only one. Living Lean is not a competition, it's a journey that should be shared to help others. Always remember that we live a life of abundance. Be generous without having an alternative motive. Help someone, just to help them. No pats on the back required. No bragging about it on social media. Just do it out of the kindness of your heart.

That's your final step to becoming a true Live Leaner.

LIVE LEAN ACTION STEPS

ACTION STEP #1: FILL UP YOUR GRATITUDE LIST

Every night before you go to bed, pull out your journal and list 5 things you've felt grateful for today. This could include the sweet taste of a fresh and juicy mango, a specific kind gesture from a friend or stranger, or hitting a new personal best at the gym. One sentence for each 5 things is all you need. This exercise is not meant to take a lot of time. It's meant to help you reflect back on the positive things that happened during your day.

1. I'm grateful for _____
2. I'm grateful for _____
3. I'm grateful for _____
4. I'm grateful for _____
5. I'm grateful for _____

When you wake up in the morning, pull out your gratitude list, and review it. It only takes 5 minutes and you will set up your mind to move toward your goals throughout the day.

ACTION STEP #2: THANK SOMEONE

Show your gratitude by thanking someone who has helped you begin your journey to Live Lean. You can do this in many different ways. Try mailing them a handwritten letter detailing what they specifically did to help you start your journey. If they live close by, you could even hand deliver it and read it to them. Or simply send an email. I personally love it when people email me their before and after transformation photos with a 1-2 sentence testimonial. I always showcase these photos on my website. I call it my Live Lean Hall of Fame because they make me so proud.

ACTION STEP #3: TEACH SOMEONE

Every time you learn something new, share it. This does not mean you should push your new Live Lean lifestyle onto your friends that are not interested in their health. I recommend you start a Facebook Fitness page, create your own blog, or starting creating a vlog. The idea is to share your journey with the universe. At first, it will seem like no one is listening, but that's ok. Just by writing about it or talking about it on camera, you are furthering your understanding of the steps to Live Lean. You could also volunteer to work with an after school program or become a "Big Brother" or "Big Sister" to someone looking for a mentor. And who knows, maybe you'll grow a following and inspire millions!

CONCLUSION

Congratulations. You've now successfully read the book. Along this journey you have been completing the necessary mindset exercises to shift your way of thinking. You now realize the power is within you. You now possess the magical recipe to the Live Lean Mindset. Be relentless. Be persistent. Believe in your abilities. Never lose focus on achieving your goals. And if you ever feel like giving up, always go back to your vision on why you desire to Live Lean.

As you progress with your Live Lean journey, every 3 months answer the following 28 questions honestly. This can give you some insight into how you're progressing towards Living Lean.

1. Did I reach the goal that I set for myself at the beginning of the year?
2. Did I complete all my workouts? Did I stick to my meal plan?
3. Did I give my best effort everyday? If not, where could I have improved?
4. Did I reach out to help someone else with something new that I learned?
5. Did I procrastinate from grocery shopping, meal planning/prep, or from completing my workouts?
6. Is my self-talk primarily a positive and re-assuring ally or did I allow negative thoughts in to cloud my actions?
7. Did my persistence overcome any self-limiting barriers that may have stopped me from working towards my goals?
8. Did I second guess why I set this goal or was I decisive in all my actions?
9. Did I allow any criticism or peer pressure from other

people stop me from taking the steps necessary to achieve my goals?

10. Did I talk negatively to myself if/when I slipped up? Or did I shake it off and keep moving forward?

11. Did I create tension with my loved ones by trying to force change on them or did I focus on leading by example?

12. Did I stay focused on my current workout program and meal plan, or did I consider switching to the latest fad/short-term plan I heard in the media?

13. Did I consider if the latest fads in nutrition and fitness on the news were from credible sources or did I make decisions based on sustainability and long-term success?

14. In what ways have I improved my daily habits to make them more efficient?

15. Did I binge on any poor food choices?

16. Did I think about my Why to overcome any potential negative urges?

17. Did I reach out to anyone in my mastermind group to give or receive help?

18. Did I truly follow my workouts as prescribed in my program or did I take shortcuts?

19. Did I take the time to plan out my meals, grocery list, and actually prepare and consume my meals as planned?

20. Did I spend excessive amounts of time watching disempowering forms of media, or did I feed my brain with positive and inspiring, mental nutrition?

21. What new ways did I find to increase my time management and productivity?

22. Did I do anything that I was not proud of?

23. How have I given extra effort even when I felt like I couldn't?

24. Have I taken the time to reward myself for all my hard work and enjoy the balance in life?

25. If I am not satisfied with my effort to date, what can I do about it to improve?

26. Do I feel like things are starting to become habits yet?

27. Am I enjoying the journey?

28. If I was the coach and I had to grade myself on my effort, what overall grade would I give myself to date?

Even though you're finished reading this book, our journey together is just starting. Rather than putting this book back on the shelf, I recommend you treat it like a study guide and review it when needed.

You are now ready to start Living Lean! Here are your next action steps so we can stay connected during your journey.

Live Lean Vow
in 186 Words

As a Live Leaner, I understand real food is my friend and not my enemy. I focus primarily on eating plants and meat, and keep sugar to a minimum. I understand protein, healthy fat, and fibrous vegetables energizes my body, ignites my metabolism, and supports recovery from my active lifestyle. I supplement when needed, but food is my main fuel source. Since balance in life is important to me, I'm not afraid to enjoy a hard-earned treat with friends. Food does not control me.

I train with intensity, sprint hard and fast, and focus on functional, compound lifts that help me become leaner, stronger, and faster at everyday tasks. Even though I'm not a high paid sports star, I realize I'm still an "athlete" at life.

And finally, I understand Living Lean is about acquiring a mindset that focuses on creating sustainable lifestyle habits and striving for consistent progress, not perfection. With this new Live Lean Mindset, I'm committed to making this my lifestyle and teaching others how to do the same.

I'm a Live Leaner and a proud member of the Live Lean Nation.

_____   _____

Signature   Date

EPILOGUE

The epilogue is the section at the end of a book that serves as the final say. So I'll end with this. You are primarily where you are today because of the choices you've made throughout your life. In this book, I've shared the exact steps for you to overcome the failure conscious mindset that is keeping you from Living Lean. If after reading this book, you still find yourself making excuses as to why you can't do it, review this section. Below, I've outlined 27 of the reasons/excuses why you may be failing to Live Lean. Remember, the power to change is inside you. One of the first steps to unlock this and take back control of your life is by first taking personal responsibility. Excuses will only give you the fuel to maintain the status quo. Your time is now.

1. YOU BLAME IT ON HAVING BAD GENETICS.

Unfortunately we can't pick our parents. Based on the luck of the draw some people are born with better genetics than others when it comes to Living Lean. Lets face it, we all have friends that can eat as many cupcakes as they want, rarely workout, yet their belt size never increases. Then there are others who seem to gain weight even just by looking at a cupcake. It sucks, but that's the way it is. Does this mean you have an excuse why you can't Live Lean? Hell no. This just means you have to hustle harder. Sorry, but it's true. You weren't dealt the hand of perfect genetics. So what. If you really want to Live Lean, you can do it. Stop blaming. Stop making excuses. Dial it in.

2. YOU DON'T HAVE A STRONG CONNECTION TO A "WHY".

If you don't have a strong emotional reason why you need to Live Lean, you've already failed. When times get tough, your

Why will be your driving factor to keep you focused. Without one, you're bound to fall back into the bad habits that got you where you currently are. Spend time on creating your Why.

3. YOU DON'T BELIEVE YOU'RE BETTER THAN AVERAGE.

This negative belief that your potential is limited will crush your ambition to raise your standard of living. Without ambition and the drive to better your life, you'll never do what is necessary to change your habits. Your potential is unlimited. Believe in yourself.

4. YOU WERE NEVER TAUGHT WHAT TO DO.

This is a simple one to overcome. Unfortunately our education system places very little resources into teaching people how to Live Lean. Fortunately, there are many resources available (like this book) that can be used to teach yourself. Remember, people get results NOT by what they know, but by how they take action on what they know. Continue to take massive action towards your goals.

5. YOU DON'T HAVE ANY SELF-DISCIPLINE.

One of the themes in this book is you will never get something for nothing. Changing your habits is inevitable. This change in lifestyle requires self-discipline and control. In a lot of ways, you are one of your greatest adversaries when it comes to Living Lean. Controlling one's self is one of the hardest things to overcome during your journey to Live Lean. It's an ongoing practice. Remember, Living Lean is about making daily progress. Not perfection.

6. YOU CAN'T AFFORD IT.

First off, Living Lean is not just for the rich. Think of it as replacing negative spending habits with positive investment habits. Money, like Living Lean, has a lot to do with mindset. Many of the steps in this book are also found in Napoleon

Hill's best-selling book, Think and Grow Rich. Why? Because achieving greatness in any aspect of life, including finance, is about mastering and controlling one's thoughts and daily actions. When you learn how to do this for your health, it can also transfer to your finances. And lets be real, when you look and feel good, you can perform at a higher level and provide more value in your chosen career. When you provide more value, you'll attract more value. Never be afraid to invest in yourself.

7. YOUR PARENTS NEVER RAISED YOU TO LIVE LEAN.

See reason #4. Just because you weren't taught something as a child, it doesn't mean you can't learn something new as an adult. You make choices everyday. Make the choice to learn and commit to replacing your negative habits with new positive habits, one day at a time.

8. YOU'LL START LIVING LEAN NEXT YEAR.

There is no perfect time to start. The only time to start Living Lean is now. Procrastination is the enemy. It's your job to acknowledge that you're using procrastination as an excuse, and take one positive action step right now to bring you closer to Living Lean.

9. YOU TRIED TO LIVE LEAN BUT A FEW BAD DAYS STOPPED YOU.

Many people start the journey to Live Lean, but few continue the journey because they lack the required persistence. Just because you had a few bad days of poor food choices and lack of movement, it doesn't mean you failed. Successful people are persistent in their actions by getting up when life knocks them down. I repeat, Living Lean is not about perfection. It's about progress. Be persistent.

10. YOU HAVE A NEGATIVE MINDSET.

Having a negative mindset will ruin all progress towards Living Lean. Don't play the role of victim. You have a choice to react to your current situation and surroundings either in a positive or negative way. I don't know of any successful person that didn't have to first overcome obstacles. Life isn't perfect. So stop wasting your energy on feeling sorry for yourself and start using it for good.

11. YOU'RE LOOKING FOR QUICK SHORTCUTS FOR FAST RESULTS.

Stop looking for shortcuts. They will always fail you. To Live Lean, you have to change your mindset, appreciate the required effort ahead of you, and put in consistent work. These behaviors will eventually translate into life-long habits. Living Lean is a process, not a quick fix. If it was, everyone would already be doing it.

12. YOU'RE JUST NOT COMMITTED TO THE PROCESS.

Have you completely committed to the decision to Live Lean? Or do you just think it would be cool to Live Lean, but you're not sure you're willing to do the necessary work. In other words, you're indecisive. Make the decision and stick to it. There's no turning back, there's no plan B, there's no option to fail.

13. YOU'RE SCARED OF THE CRITICISM FROM YOUR FRIENDS.

In other words, peer pressure. Remember when Johnny made fun of you for not wanting to smoke that cigarette in high school? It made you feel less of a person right? Well now that you're an adult, your friends are probably still peer pressuring you into drinking excessively and eating belly busting foods. Once again, it all comes down to choices. Be strong. You're in control of what you do and don't do.

14. YOUR HUSBAND/WIFE DOESN'T WANT TO LIVE LEAN.

Unfortunately this is a tough one. The person you've committed your life to doesn't share the same vision or goals that you do. In fact, in many ways it may seem like they're taking you further away from your goals. Refer to what we discussed earlier. Lead with actions, not with words. Eventually they should come around. Also, remember that even though you do many things together, you don't have to do EVERYTHING together. It's okay and it's even very healthy for couples to have separate hobbies and separate goals.

15. YOU SUFFER FROM "ANALYSIS PARALYSIS".

We are inundated with information on how to lose weight. Unfortunately for some, this over consumption of information can lead to confusion and the dreaded case of "analysis paralysis". Simply put, you won't make a decision or take any action because you're overwhelmed with what to do first. Inevitably, this leads you to not taking any action at all. Find one mentor that is getting the results that you want and forget about what all the other "experts" are saying. Follow this mentors advice, and take it one step at a time.

16. YOU SURROUND YOURSELF WITH THE WRONG PEOPLE.

As the saying goes, you live up to, or in most cases, down to the 5 people you hang out with most. Next time you're out, take a look at another group of friends. More likely than not, they'd all be similar in size and shape. If you're currently out of shape but are still the healthiest member of your friends, it's time to expand your circle.

17. YOU STRIVE FOR PERFECTION.

Again, Living Lean is not about perfection. It's about continuous progress. In fact, striving for perfection can be the enemy of Living Lean. It's not an all or nothing approach.

Focus on doing the right things the majority of the time. Everything else will eventually work out.

18. YOU DON'T ENJOY WORKING OUT OR EATING BORING FOODS.

People get this one wrong all the time. Let me be clear. Living Lean is NOT about spending your life in the gym and eating nothing but chicken and broccoli. That is not a sustainable lifestyle. Living Lean is all about creating life-long habits. Trust me, with the right plan, you can make healthy food taste great. You can make your workouts enjoyable. It's a learning process, but it's all a part of the journey. My life is living proof that it's possible. I love and enjoy every single bite I eat and look forward to the challenge of my workouts.

19. YOU LACK THE CONCENTRATION TO FOCUS. YOU PREFER FOLLOWING SEXY SHORT-TERM TRENDS/FADS RATHER THAN PROVEN STEPS THAT WORK FOREVER.

For example, you quit your current program to start the next quick-fix fad program that promises you faster results. Or you hear about a liquid diet that promises you to lose 10 pounds in one week. It's easy to fall into the trap of fads and trends. Very rarely, especially in the health industry, are these trends sustainable. This lack of focus ruins progress. The Live Lean steps are sustainable because they form into habits. Stop chasing shortcuts and focus on the end goal of creating sustainable healthy habits. Focus and trust the process.

20. YOU CONTINUALLY GIVE IN TO YOUR "PERCEIVED" CRAVINGS.

Many people declare themselves as having a sweet tooth. They believe it's just "who they are". Wrong mindset. We all crave things in life. The difference between those who are Living Lean and those who are not, is the mindset towards those things. Just because you think you want something, it doesn't mean your body actually needs it. Crave health not junk.

21. YOU AREN'T ENTHUSIASTIC ABOUT LIVING LEAN.

Living Lean is simple but NOT easy. Things that are simple to do means they're just as simple NOT to do. Those who are successful at Living Lean are enthusiastic and open to the lifestyle changes required.

22. YOU'RE CLOSED-MINDED.

Although it's important to stay focused on the fitness, nutrition, and mindset steps to Live Lean, we must keep an open mind. The science of nutrition in particular, is constantly evolving. This doesn't mean you need to read research studies, but it does mean you need to keep an open mind to the changing times. For example, egg yolks were once thought to be the devil. We now know egg yolks are awesome for our health. Don't be closed-minded. Remain open.

23. YOU TRY TO DO IT ALL BY YOURSELF.

Invest in yourself. Don't be afraid to spend money on a well designed workout program, nutrition plan, cookbook, etc. from qualified people that you trust. When you put some skin in the game (i.e. money), you're much more likely to take action on the investment than if you go at it blindly.

24. YOU TAKE ADVICE FROM THE WRONG PEOPLE.

Would you take advice on how to get rich from someone who is bankrupt? I hope not. So why would you take advice from someone who is not Living Lean. Invest in the help of those that are not only getting the results you want but they are also getting other people the same results as well.

25. YOU'RE NOT BEING HONEST WITH YOURSELF.

Many people are dishonest to themselves. They convince themselves that they are trying hard, but deep down they know they're just staying inside their comfort zone. Living Lean is about getting outside of that comfort zone. It's about stretching your limits and raising your life's standards. Take a hard look at yourself and ask, am I truly giving it my all or could I take it to the next level.

26. YOU'RE DOING IT FOR THE WRONG REASONS.

Living Lean is not just about getting abs. Abs are just a by-product. Living Lean is about gaining the self-confidence to be comfortable in your own skin. It provides a sense of empowerment that if you can transform your body, you can transform any part of your life. Go deeper with your Why. It shouldn't just be about the vanity.

27. YOU DON'T HAVE ENOUGH TIME.

Everyone has 24 hours in a day and tens of thousands of people are enjoying a workout right now as you read these words. You can't create more time. But you can manage your time more effectively. When you understand your Why, you make the principles of Living Lean a priority in your life. Once you re-focus your time and priorities, finding 45 minutes in the day to workout won't seem impossible.

Now that you've reviewed the above list, go ahead and highlight which ones you're currently failing at. Be honest with yourself. Once you do that, review the list with someone who knows you well. Have them go through the 27 reasons and highlight those that they think you're failing at. Be sure to make the person comfortable with being honest with you. Many times we may not see what others see about ourselves. This makes it a very important exercise to see how others perceive you. Do not get offended or take this feedback as an attack. Use this feedback to inspire your growth.

As you've been learning throughout this book, many of these failures come down to having a negative mindset. That is why this book was created. It serves as the missing link to provide people with the necessary principles and action steps to overcome each of these mindset failures.

Next Steps:

#1. Download our FREE Ultimate Live Leaner Starter Guide:

I created something very special for you over at my blog, LiveLeanTV.com. For a limited time, I'm giving away my Ultimate Live Lean Starter Guide for FREE. This starter guide will show you exactly how to start Living Lean in 30 days or less. It includes a 4-week "Hot Body" workout program, a weekly meal plan, cooking lesson recipe videos for each meal inside the meal plan, and a grocery list featuring all the ingredients to make the meals. It's all done for you and is 100% **FREE**. To download this limited time only starter guide,

go to:

Ultimate Live Lean Starter Guide:

http://www.LiveLeanTV.com/free-stuff

#2. Subscribe to our Live Lean TV Show:

Never miss an episode of Live Lean TV by subscribing to our show on YouTube. This is where we share all the best fitness and nutrition tips, workouts, and motivational videos to Live Lean 365 days a year.

Subscribe on YouTube: http://www.youtube.com/ LiveLeanTV

#3. Follow for more daily motivation:

Be sure to stop by my social media channels and say hi. You could also be a little less formal and say something like, "What up bro, loved your Think and Live Lean book, you're like totally awesome man". Your call.

Follow me here:

Facebook: http://www.facebook.com/bradgouthrofitness

Instagram: http://www.instagram.com/bradgouthro

Twitter: http://www.twitter.com/bradgouthro

Snapchat: BradGouthro

#4. Final Step. Sign the Live Lean Vow.

Start changing your life
at TeamLiveLean.com

Get unlimited access to tools, exclusive members-only content, plus Brad's proven diet and fitness program so you can:
✓ Harness your power to Live Lean
✓ Lose Weight
✓ Build Strength
✓ Get Healthy

At TeamLiveLean.com you'll get:

- A brand new exclusive monthly training program every month
- A brand new exclusive video cooking lesson every week
- A weekly meal plan and grocery list
- Access to Brad, Jessica, & our community of like-minded individuals
- Lifetime 20% off discount on all new Live Lean digital programs

Claim your membership now at TeamLiveLean.com.

Use coupon code: thinkandlivelean
for 50% off the 1st month

This is the perfect companion to your new book!